OPHTHALMOLOGY FOR PRIMARY CARE

Gloria Wu, MD

Assistant Surgeon
Massachusetts Eye and Ear Infirmary
Clinical Instructor
Harvard Medical School
Associate Clinical Professor
Tufts University School of Medicine
Boston, Massachusetts

OPHTHALMOLOGY FOR PRIMARY CARE

W.B. SAUNDERS COMPANY
A Division of Harcourt Brace & Company
Philadelphia   London   Toronto   Montreal   Sydney   Tokyo

W.B. SAUNDERS COMPANY
A Division of Harcourt Brace & Company

The Curtis Center
Independence Square West
Philadelphia, Pennsylvania 19106

Library of Congress Cataloging-in-Publication Data

Wu, Gloria.
Ophthalmology for primary care / Gloria Wu.—1st ed.

p.   cm.

ISBN 0–7216–5078–3

1. Eye—Diseases.   2. Primary care (Medicine)   I. Title. [DNLM: 1. Eye
    Diseases—diagnosis.   2. Eye Diseases—therapy. WW 141 W958o 1997]

RE46.W977 1997   617.7—dc21

DNLM/DLC   96–49580

OPHTHALMOLOGY FOR PRIMARY CARE   ISBN 0–7216–5078–3

Printed in the United States of America.

Last digit is the print number: 9   8   7   6   5   4   3   2   1

To my daughters, Margaret and Catherine,
to my husband, Paul,
and to my parents.

Preface

This book is written for the busy primary care physician who encounters common eye complaints. The main goal is to answer questions about ophthalmology in an out-patient setting for primary care physicians, general internists, family practitioners, and residents. Nurses, nurse practitioners, physician assistants, emergency medical technicians, and medical students will find the book useful, as well. The intention of the book is to make ophthalmology accessible to all branches of primary care.

The book provides an overview of the anatomy of the eye, examination techniques, and common eye disorders such as myopia, lid growths, contact lens problems, and ocular infections. Topics described in more detail include sudden visual loss, eye emergencies associated with pain and visual loss, including glaucoma, and optic nerve disorders such as optic disc edema and papilledema. The chapter on systemic disease delineates important ophthalmic features of diabetes, hypertension, AIDS, and neoplastic conditions. Although tumors of the eye and the ocular tissues are rare, the more common entities are included. There is a chapter on the pediatric examination and the common eye disorders in children. The last chapter is a summary of ocular emergencies for quick reference. An explanation of the ophthalmologist's note, common eye medications, and the routine tests performed in an ophthalmologist's office are presented in the appendix.

I hope that my non-ophthalmic colleagues will find this book useful in their everyday practice, and that it reinforces continued dialogue between ophthalmologists and internal medicine and primary care colleagues.

Gloria Wu, MD

Acknowledgments

First and foremost, I would like to acknowledge the superb teaching of D. Jackson Coleman, M.D., Chairman of the Department of Ophthalmology at New York Hospital-Cornell Medical Center, where I trained as a resident. In addition, I would like to thank Drs. Dianne Aronian, Peter Odell, Walter Peretz, Peter Laino, Wayne Whitmore, Barrett Haik, David Abramson, Edward Cotlier, and the late Robert Ellsworth, who taught me the art and science of ophthalmology when I was a young resident.

I would like to thank the ophthalmologists and primary care practitioners at St. Elizabeth's Medical Center, Newton-Wellesley Hospital, Norwood Hospital, Tufts-New England Medical Center, New England Deaconess Hospital, New England Baptist Hospital, Beth Israel Medical Center, and Brigham and Women's Hospital for allowing me the privilege of taking care of their patients.

For the past 10 years, I have had the honor of teaching the residents rotating through the emergency room and the general eye service at the Massachusetts Eye and Ear Infirmary. I would like to thank the emergency room staff, most notably, Ms. Terri Kunzweiler, Director of Emergency Room Nursing, Dr. Mary Gilbert Lawrence and Dr. Ted Murphy, Directors of the General Eye Service. As one of the clinical attendings at the Massachusetts Eye and Ear Infirmary, I am grateful for the support of our chief, Dr. Frederick Jakobiec.

For the actual compilation of the manuscript, I would like to acknowledge the expert organizational and technical skills of Monal Shah, Cristina Hernandez, Rene Bonin, Sarah Wilson, Renee Thorn, Nancy Sacco, Dianne Connelly, Sara Zekri, Irwin Sterbakov, Kim Fletcher, Anna Moon, and Tammy Tam. During the year that I spent writing the manuscript, Richard Lampert of W.B. Saunders provided attentive editorial guidance.

I am grateful for the privilege of serving my patients. Their questions have continued to motivate us, as physicians, to find the answers.

Lastly, I would like to thank my husband and my children for their enthusiastic support throughout this project.

Gloria Wu, MD

Contents

Chapter 1   **Anatomy of the Eye**   1

Chapter 2   **Examination Techniques**   7

Chapter 3   **Common Eye Disorders**   17

Chapter 4   **Sudden Visual Loss**   63

Chapter 5   **Eye Emergencies Associated with Pain and Vision Loss**   77

Chapter 6   **Systemic Disease**   95

Chapter 7   **Optic Nerve Disorders**   131

Chapter 8   **Primary Tumors of the Eye**   147

Chapter 9   **Examination of the Pediatric Patient**   159

Chapter 10   **Ophthalmic Emergencies**   171

Appendix   177

Index   193

Color Plates Follow Contents

Color Plates

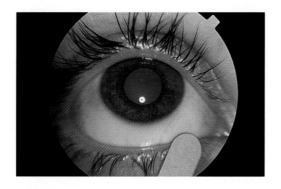

• **FIGURE 2–5**
Inferior cul de sac and fluorescein strip.

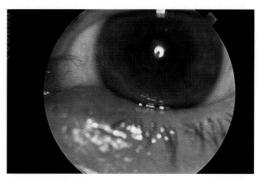

• **FIGURE 3–3**
Chalazion.

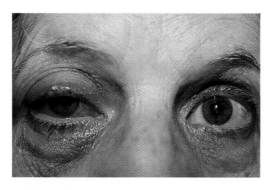

• **FIGURE 3–4**
Preseptal cellulitis.

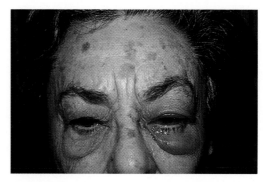

• **FIGURE 3–5**
Orbital cellulitis.

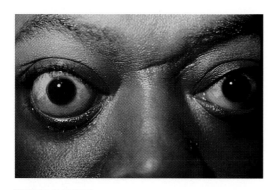

• **FIGURE 3–7**
Graves' disease with unequal edema of the eyelids.

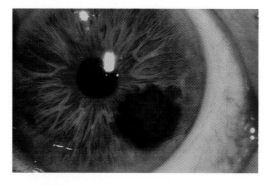

• **FIGURE 3–15**
Iris nevus.

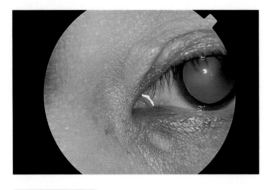

• **FIGURE 3–16**
Xanthelasma.

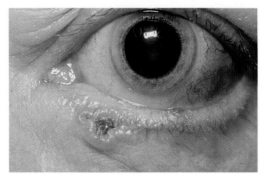

• **FIGURE 3–18**
Basal cell carcinoma. (Courtesy of Peter Rubin, MD, Boston, MA.)

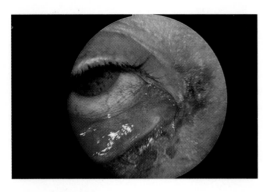

• **FIGURE 3–19**
Squamous cell carcinoma.

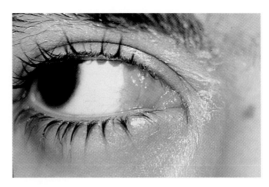

• **FIGURE 3–20**
Lymphoma of the medial canthus.

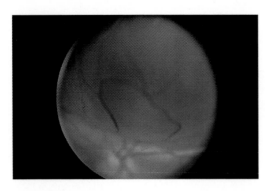

• **FIGURE 3–21**
Malignant melanoma.

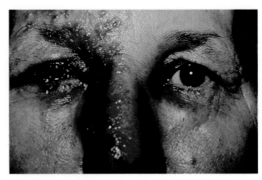

• **FIGURE 3–23**
Herpes zoster conjunctivitis.

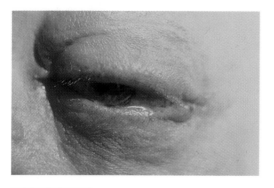

• **FIGURE 3–24**
Gonorrheal conjunctivitis with purulence.

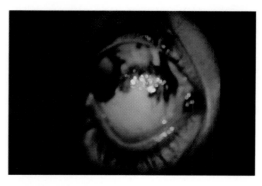

• **FIGURE 3–26**
Conjunctival melanoma.

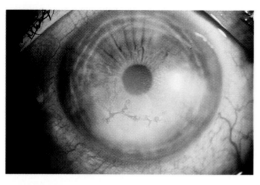

• **FIGURE 3–29**
Dendrite in herpes simplex keratitis. (From
American Academy of Ophthalmology. External
Disease and Cornea: A Multimedia Collection.
San Francisco, 1994)

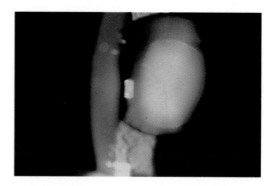

• **FIGURE 3–35**
Cataract.

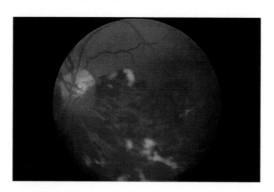

• **FIGURE 4–2**
Branch retinal vein occlusion.

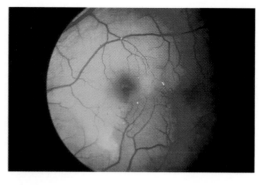

• **FIGURE 4–3**
Central retinal artery occlusion.

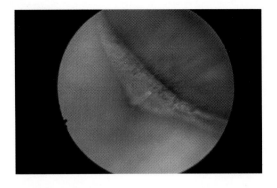

• FIGURE 4–5
Area of the pars plana in relation to that of the retina.

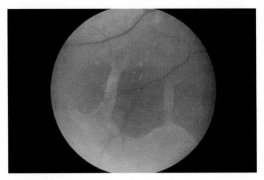

• FIGURE 4–8
Retinal detachment.

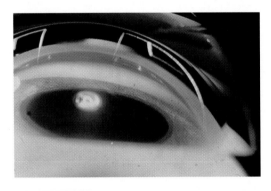

• FIGURE 5–2
Angle of the eye with fine neovascularization.

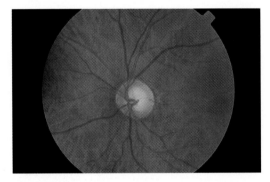

• FIGURE 5–3
Typical glaucomatous cupping. Note the hallowed-out appearance of the optic disc except for the thin border.

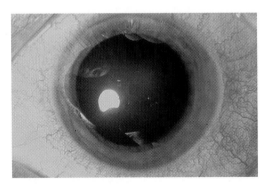

• FIGURE 5–7
Conjunctival injection from contact lens overwear.

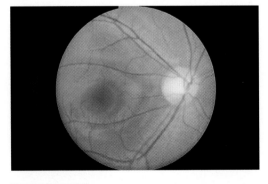

• FIGURE 5–8
Retinal edema from blunt trauma to the eye.

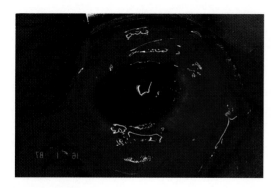

• FIGURE 5–9
Ruptured globe.

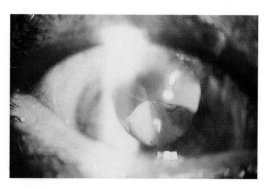

• FIGURE 5–10
Extruded lens in a ruptured globe resulting from severe trauma to the eye. (Courtesy of Lory Snady-McCoy, MD, Providence, RI.)

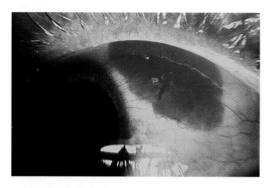

• FIGURE 5–11
Scleral laceration from penetrating injury.

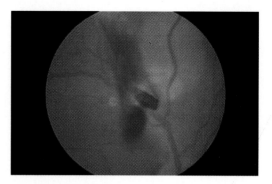

• FIGURE 5–12
Penetrating injury to the eye with intraocular metallic foreign body lodged in the retina.

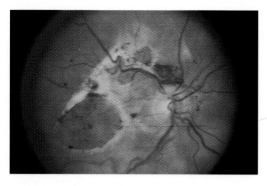

• FIGURE 5–13
Scarring of the retina caused by blunt trauma to the eye.

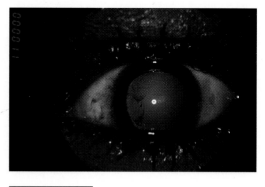

• FIGURE 5–14
Blood in the anterior chamber and glaucoma from traumatic injury to the globe.

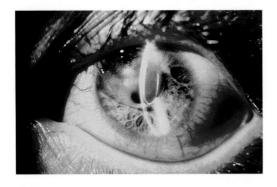

• **FIGURE 6–1**
Iris atrophy.

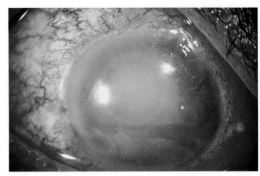

• **FIGURE 6–2**
Neovascular glaucoma.

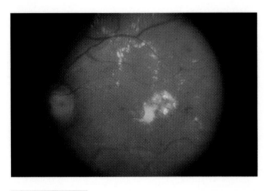

• **FIGURE 6–3**
Hard exudate from diabetic retinopathy.

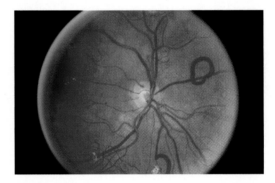

• **FIGURE 6–4**
Venous loop.

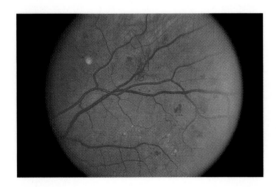

• **FIGURE 6–5**
Retinal neovascularization.

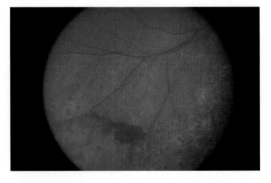

• **FIGURE 6–7**
Vitreous hemorrhage.

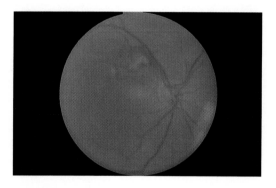

• FIGURE 6–8
Cotton wool spot.

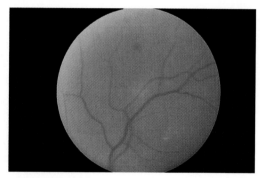

• FIGURE 6–9
Dot hemorrhage in background diabetic retinopathy.

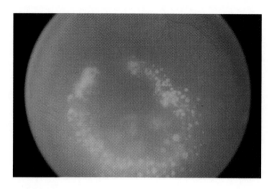

• FIGURE 6–10
Hard exudates.

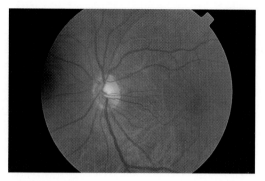

• FIGURE 6–11
No diabetic retinopathy.

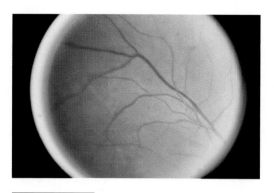

• FIGURE 6–12
Background diabetic retinopathy with fewer than 30 microaneurysms.

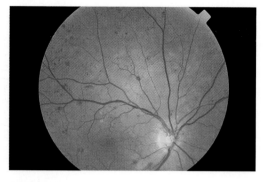

• FIGURE 6–13
Nonproliferative diabetic retinopathy.

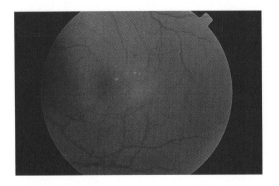

• FIGURE 6–14
Mild diabetic macular edema.

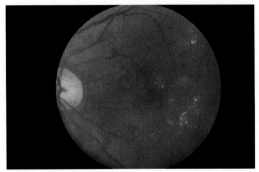

• FIGURE 6–15
Diabetic macular edema, with changes associated with nonproliferative diabetic retinopathy.

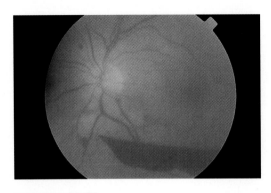

• FIGURE 6–16
Diabetic vitreous hemorrhage.

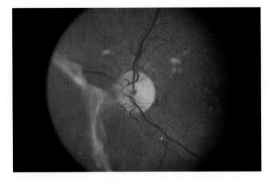

• FIGURE 6–17
Mild diabetic traction retinal detachment.

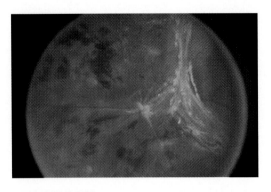

• FIGURE 6–18
Severe diabetic traction retinal detachment.

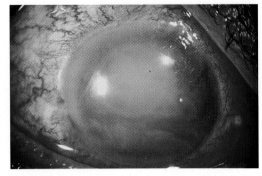

• FIGURE 6–21
New vessels on the iris and hyphema in the anterior chamber.

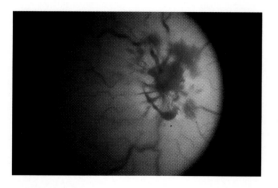

• FIGURE 6–25
Optic nerve hemorrhage in acute lymphocytic
leukemia.

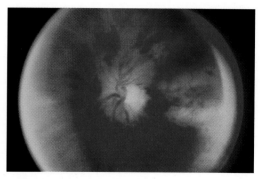

• FIGURE 6–26
Retinal hemorrhages in acute lymphocytic
leukemia.

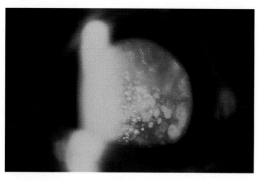

• FIGURE 6–27
Vitreous infiltrates in acute lymphocytic leukemia.

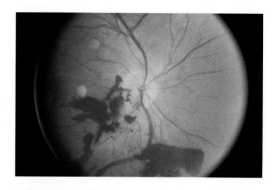

• FIGURE 6–28
Retinal hemorrhages in Hodgkin's lymphoma.

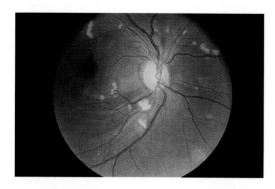

• FIGURE 6–29
Cotton wool spots in acquired immunodeficiency syndrome.

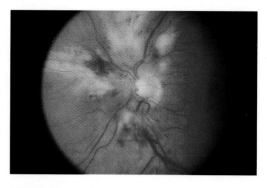

• FIGURE 6–30
Cytomegalovirus retinitis with cotton wool spots.

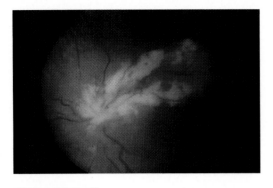

• FIGURE 6–31
Cytomegalovirus retinitis with necrosis along the vasculature.

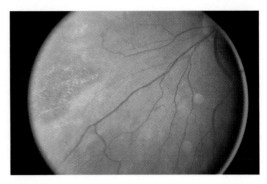

• FIGURE 6–32
Regressed cytomegalovirus retinitis.

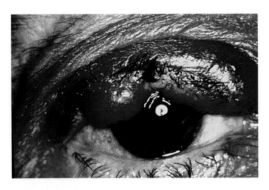

• FIGURE 6–33
Kaposi's sarcoma.

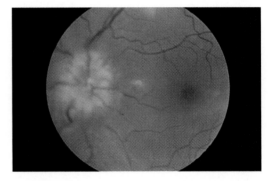

• FIGURE 6–34
Optic nerve edema with associated cotton wool spots in acquired immunodeficiency syndrome.

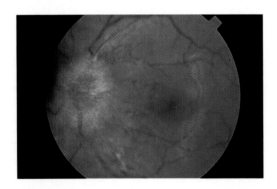

• FIGURE 7–1
Papilledema.

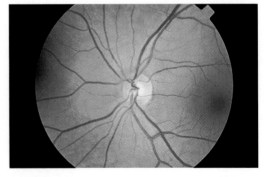

• FIGURE 7–2
Optic neuritis.

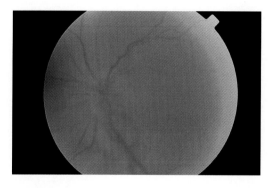

• FIGURE 7–3
Anterior ischemic optic neuropathy.

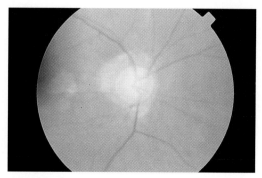

• FIGURE 7–4
Optic atrophy.

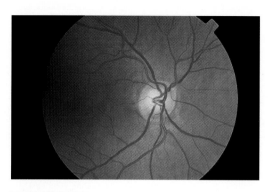

• FIGURE 7–5
Temporal arteritis.

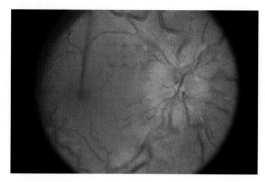

• FIGURE 7–6
Optic disc edema in Lyme disease.

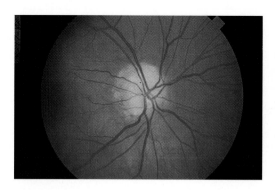

• FIGURE 7–7
Drusen of the optic nerve, showing nodular formation of the optic nerve head.

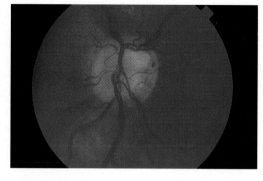

• FIGURE 7–8
Drusen of the optic nerve, showing displacement and gliosis of the overlying optic nerve vessels.

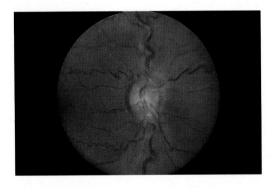

• FIGURE 7–9
Optic disc edema in malignant hypertension.

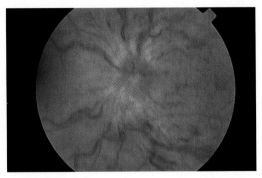

• FIGURE 7–10
Papillophlebitis.

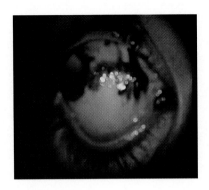

• FIGURE 8–4
Melanoma of the conjunctiva.

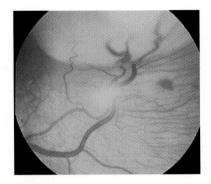

• FIGURE 8–5
Retinoblastoma.

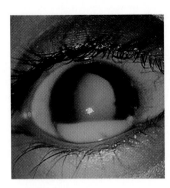

• FIGURE 8–6
Leukokoria (white reflex) and
hypopon in a child with
retinoblastoma.

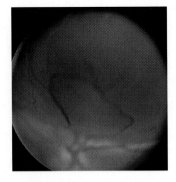

• FIGURE 8–7
Malignant melanoma of the
choroid.

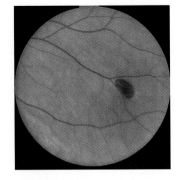

• FIGURE 8–8
Choroidal nevus, which can
be confused with malignant
melanoma of the choroid.

1

Anatomy of the Eye

SURFACE ANATOMY

The eye is framed by the eyebrows and the area of the skin called the *orbit* (Fig. 1–1). The eye is protected by the upper and lower eyelids. The underside of the eyelid is called the *tarsus*. The eyelashes are called *cilia*. Next to the cilia are little openings of glands called the *orifices of the meibomian glands*. The nasal aspect of the eye is called the *medial canthus*, and the far temporal area of the eyelids is called the *lateral canthus*. In the medial canthal area are the *lacrimal caruncle* and the *lacrimal punctum*: two puncta are in each eye—the *upper punctum* and the *lower punctum* (Fig. 1–2). An additional fold exists called the *plica semilunaris*. This area is usually referred to as the *adnexa oculi* (Figs. 1–1 and 1–2; Table 1–1).

The white part of the eye is called the *sclera*. The sclera is covered by a clear translucent tissue called the *conjunctiva* (Fig. 1–1). The clear part of the eye is the *cornea*. It protects the inner structures of the eye (Fig. 1–1). The intersection of the sclera and cornea is called the *limbus* (Table 1–2).

The *iris* is the part of the eye that has color, such as blue and green. The iris is made up of two muscles that work to dilate and constrict the pupil. Within the iris are radial muscle fibers and circular muscle fibers.

The circular iris defines the pupil. The size of the pupil can vary with age, nearsightedness, light, and accommodation (Fig. 1–1).

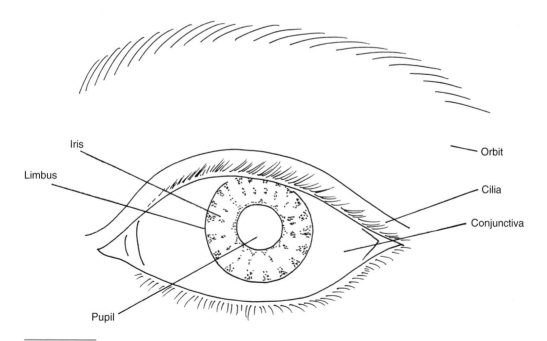

• **FIGURE 1–1**
The eye.

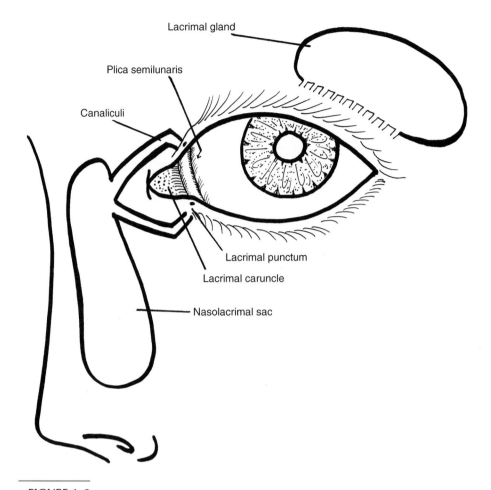

• **FIGURE 1–2**
The external eye.

TABLE 1–1
ANATOMY OF THE EXTERNAL EYE

Orbit
Eyebrows
Eyelids
Tarsus (connective tissue plate of upper and lower eyelids)
Cilia or eyelashes
Meibomian glands (glands that nourish the cilia; their glandular openings are next to the cilia)
Lacrimal caruncle (fleshy area in the medial aspect of the eyelids that houses the lacrimal puncta)
Lacrimal puncta (the entrance of the nasolacrimal system, one of the drainage sites for tears. Tears are directed toward the puncta by capillary attraction and gravity and by the blinking action of the eyelids. This causes tears to flow down into the nasolacrimal duct into the nose)
Plica semilunaris (a semicircular fold in the medial part of the eye)

TABLE 1–2
ANATOMY OF THE GLOBE

Conjunctiva (clear translucent tissue covering of the white sclera. The conjunctiva becomes edematous or erythematous in various infections, e.g., conjunctivitis)
Sclera (white ocular coat of the eye. It is made of collagenous connective tissue)
Cornea (clear part of the eye)
Limbus (the intersection of the cornea with the sclera)
Iris (the blue- or brown-colored part of the eye. It can sometimes show a mixture of colors. Occasionally, patients exhibit a blue eye and a brown eye—iris heterochromia)
Pupil (the central opening of the eye. The iris forms this centrally placed aperture of the eye, the pupil)

ANATOMY OF THE INTERNAL EYE STRUCTURES
(Table 1–3)

Under the cornea is the *anterior chamber*. In this area, clear fluid called the *aqueous* bathes the structures in the eye with vitamin C, electrolytes, and oxygen. In this area, release of cellular debris or macrophages can occur, depending on the disease process. The aqueous is formed in the area called the *ciliary body*, which is located on the underside of the iris (Fig. 1–3).

As the cornea meets the iris, a space called the *angle* is created. This area houses the *trabecular meshwork*, which drains the eye of aqueous every 20 minutes. Degenerative damage to the trabecular meshwork can occur over time, leading to problems with the regular and timely drainage of the aqueous. This is one of the mechanisms of glaucoma, the leading cause of blindness for all ages in America. The trabecular meshwork drains its aqueous via Schlemm's canal, which is part of the venous drainage of the eye.

Under the iris is the *lens*, which is tethered into place by diaphanous

TABLE 1–3
INTERNAL STRUCTURES OF THE EYE

Cornea
Anterior chamber (the space between the cornea and the iris)
Angle (in the area of the limbus, where the cornea and the iris form an "angle," is the area that houses the drainage system for the aqueous)
Trabecular meshwork (the drainage system for the aqueous)
Schlemm's canal (the trabecular meshwork drains into Schlemm's canal, which in turn drains into the venous system of the eye)
Ciliary body (a continuation of the iris that creates the liquid aqueous)
Zonules (fibrils that hold the lens in place)
Lens
Pars plana (the continuation of the retina as it approaches anteriorly)
Retina
Choroid (vascular tissue of the globe)
Optic nerve

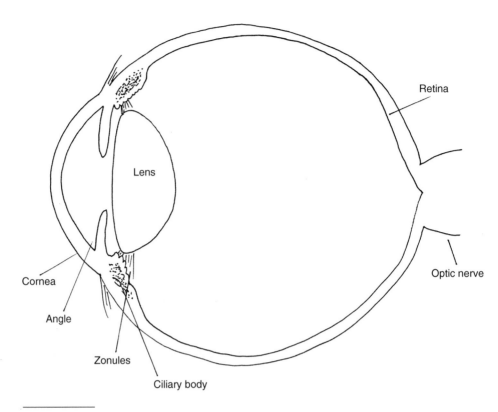

• **FIGURE 1–3**
The eye in cross-section.

ligaments called *zonules* at the level of the ciliary body. The end of the ciliary body meets the *pars plana*, which is the beginning of the *retina*. The retina is the inside lining of the eye. It is made of 10 cell layers measuring 350 μm in thickness. The sclera, seen at the surface of the eye, continues posteriorly to form the outermost layer in this region. The layer of sclera is made of white connective tissue. Between the retina and the sclera is the vascular layer called the *choroid*, which is composed of sheets of blood vessels. The posterior aspect of the globe is the *optic nerve*, which provides the connection to the brain (Fig. 1–3).

2

Examination
Techniques

WHO SHOULD UNDERGO ANNUAL EYE EXAMINATIONS

We suggest that yearly eye examinations be performed for patients older than 40 years to test for visual acuity, glaucoma and to examine the optic nerve. In patients with hypertension or diabetes, examination of the optic nerve and eyegrounds, as can be performed with the direct ophthalmoscope, should occur more frequently. For these patients, a yearly examination of the retina by the ophthalmologist is recommended (Tables 2–1 and 2–2). The rest of the chapters in this book deal with specific eye problems.

EQUIPMENT IN THE PRIMARY CARE OFFICE SETTING
(Table 2–3)

Snellen Visual Acuity Chart: Wall Chart and Near Card

Visual acuity measurement is an important indicator of the extent of the eye problem. The *Snellen visual acuity chart* is the "E chart" seen commonly in most physicians' offices. It can be readily obtained through medical equipment and optical companies. The line "20/20" defines the line read by average normal people at 20 feet from the chart (6/6 is the metric equivalent). The line read by average normal people at 400 feet is 20/400 (Fig. 2–1, Table 2–1).

The patient's right eye should be tested first, then the left eye. The patient should always be asked to wear his or her spectacles so that the best result is obtained.

The patient faces the chart at a distance of 20 feet, covers the left eye, and has the right eye open to read the chart. The same procedure is repeated, with the right eye occluded. The patient reads successively smaller lines. Physicians should determine the smallest possible line that the patient can read.

A near card can be used to test a patient who is wearing the glasses he or she usually wears for reading. Again, one eye is covered at a time. The card is usually held 16 inches away from the patient. A ruler can be used to measure the distance, or a 16-inch piece of string can be attached to the near card (Fig. 2–2).

Pinhole

A *pinhole* is a small device that allows the physician to see if refractive error is the cause of the patient's decreased vision. The device can be obtained at any optical house. The patient is asked to look through this device and ascertain if his or her visual acuity improves. If so, the patient needs a change in his or her eyeglass prescription. If no improvement can be obtained, the

TABLE 2–1

WHAT IS THE BASIC EYE EXAMINATION?

1. Snellen visual acuity chart (distance or near visual acuity, preferably both).

2. Pupillary examination.

3. Optic nerve evaluation with the hand-held direct ophthalmoscope.

TABLE 2–2

WHO SHOULD HAVE AN EYE EXAMINATION?

Patients older than 40 years of age: to evaluate visual acuity, test for glaucoma, and evaluate the optic nerve.
Patients who have hypertension, diabetes, or thyroid disease: to evaluate visual acuity and test for hypertensive retinopathy, diabetic retinopathy, and thyroid eye disease.
Patients who complain of visual loss.
Children who are about to enter school.

TABLE 2–3

WHAT EQUIPMENT IS NECESSARY FOR THE BASIC EYE EXAMINATION?

Snellen visual acuity chart (Snellen wall chart for distance visual acuity and Snellen visual acuity near card)
Pinhole (optional)
Penlight
Fluorescein strips (to detect corneal abrasions in the emergency room setting)
Direct ophthalmoscope

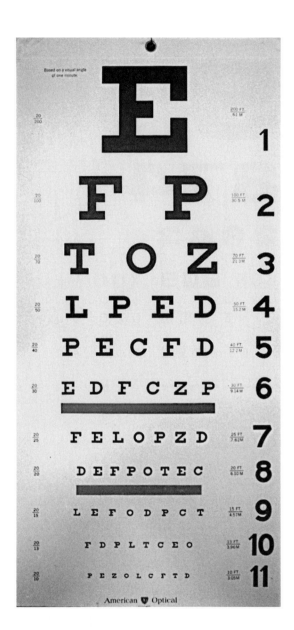

• **FIGURE 2–1**
Visual acuity chart. (Photography by Michele Macrakis.)

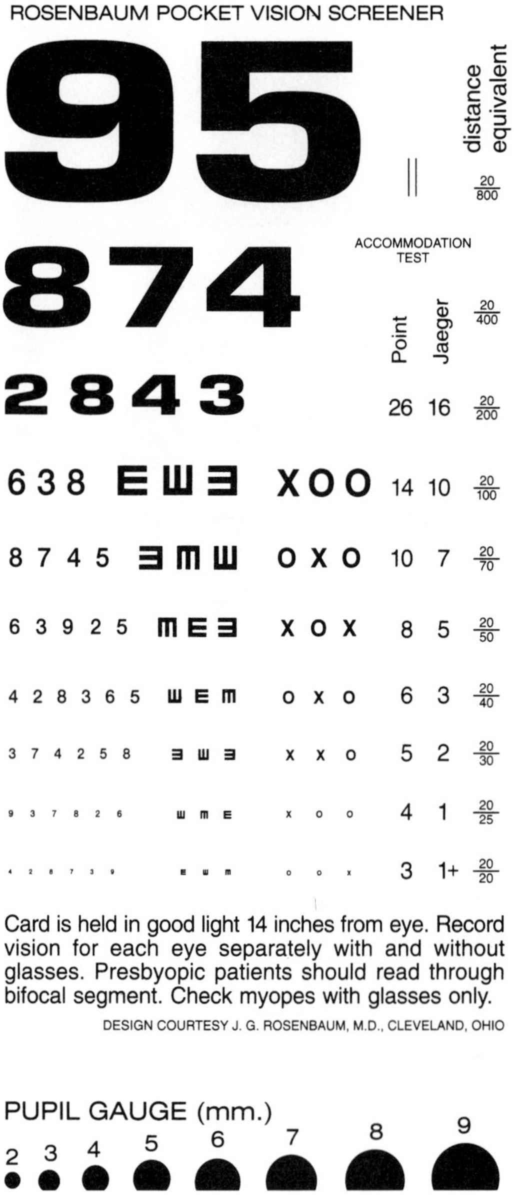

ROSENBAUM POCKET VISION SCREENER

		Point	Jaeger	distance equivalent
95				$\frac{20}{800}$
874	ACCOMMODATION TEST			$\frac{20}{400}$
2 8 4 3		26	16	$\frac{20}{200}$
6 3 8 **E Ш Ǝ** X O O		14	10	$\frac{20}{100}$
8 7 4 5 **Ǝ ɯ Ш** O X O		10	7	$\frac{20}{70}$
6 3 9 2 5 **ɯ E Ǝ** X O X		8	5	$\frac{20}{50}$
4 2 8 3 6 5 Ш E ɯ O X O		6	3	$\frac{20}{40}$
3 7 4 2 5 8 Ǝ Ш Ǝ X X O		5	2	$\frac{20}{30}$
9 3 7 8 2 6 Ш ɯ E X O O		4	1	$\frac{20}{25}$
4 2 8 7 3 9 E Ш ɯ O O X		3	1+	$\frac{20}{20}$

Card is held in good light 14 inches from eye. Record vision for each eye separately with and without glasses. Presbyopic patients should read through bifocal segment. Check myopes with glasses only.

DESIGN COURTESY J. G. ROSENBAUM, M.D., CLEVELAND, OHIO

PUPIL GAUGE (mm.)

2 3 4 5 6 7 8 9

• **FIGURE 2–2**
Near visual acuity card.

patient may have another problem that necessitates referral to an ophthal-mologist or eye care specialist (Fig. 2–3).

Penlight

The *penlight* allows the physician to look into the external eye structures. For instance, the penlight distinguishes whether the eyelid or the eyeball is the problem.

The penlight allows for the examination of the pupils in the swinging flashlight test. It tests the ability of the pupils to constrict and therefore the functioning of the third cranial nerve.

With the flashlight, the physician can also ask the patient to look to the right and to the left, testing the third and sixth cranial nerves. In addition,

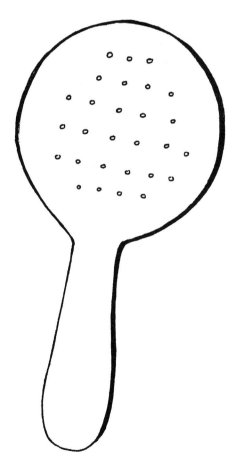

• **FIGURE 2–3**
Pinhole assessment tool.

with the patient looking downward and right and downward and left, the superior oblique muscle, and cranial nerve IV, can be tested (Fig. 2–4).

Fluorescein Strips

Fluorescein strips are specially coated strips of filter paper that are readily available at optical supply houses. They reveal corneal abrasions or any disruption in the cornea by staining bright green. This tool enables the physician to make a quick diagnosis of eye pain in patients with contact lens problems or foreign body sensation in the eye (Fig. 2–5; see also Fig. 2–5 Color Plate 1).

The patient is instructed to look upward, gently lower the lower lid of the eye, and place the test strip in the inferior cul de sac (Fig. 2–5; see also Fig. 2–5 Color Plate 1) (see Treatment for Corneal Abrasion, Chapter 3).

Direct Ophthalmoscope

The *direct ophthalmoscope* in the primary care physician's office can be used to detect important ocular diagnoses, such as glaucoma, diabetic

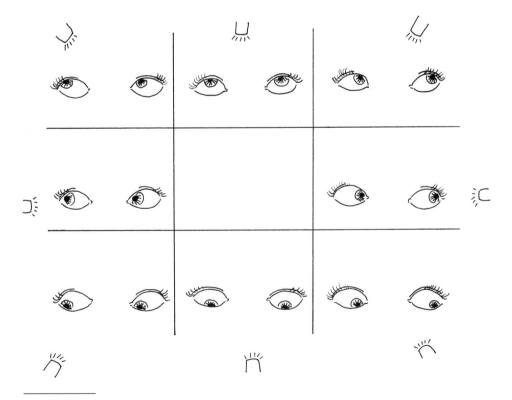

• **FIGURE 2–4**
Penlight examination.

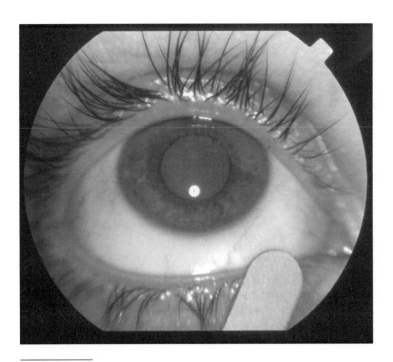

• **FIGURE 2–5**
Inferior cul de sac and fluorescein strip.

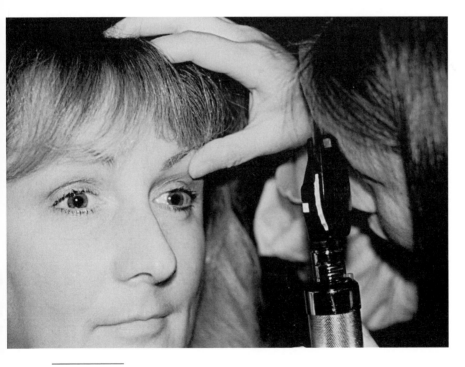

• **FIGURE 2–6**
Physician using direct ophthalmoscope to examine a patient.

retinopathy, hypertension, optic disc edema, papilledema, and cataract (Fig. 2–6). The direct ophthalmoscope allows a view into the patient's retina and optic nerve; it provides a wealth of information.

The direct ophthalmoscope should be held at the patient's eye level, at an angle of 30 degrees. The physician examiner wears his or her own glasses while performing this examination, or the physician dials his or her own prescription into the direct ophthalmoscope before starting the examination.

In examining the patient's right eye, the physician approaches from the patient's right side and uses the physician's right eye to look inside. If the physician is examining the patient's left eye, the physician approaches from the patient's left side and uses the physician's left eye to look inside. In this fashion, the physician avoids the patient's nose in the examination process. The examination is begun at the high plus numbers (black digits) and progresses downward to zero so that the examiner's eye is in focus with the patient's retina. At a 6-inch viewing distance, the high plus numbers on the ophthalmoscope dial enable the examiner to see any lens changes or cataracts. At a closer viewing distance, with the direct ophthalmoscope setting of zero, the physician is focused on the patient's retina.

3

Common Eye Disorders

NEARSIGHTEDNESS (MYOPIA), FARSIGHTEDNESS (HYPEROPIA), AND PRESBYOPIA

Nearsightedness, or Myopia

The light rays entering a long eye cause the point of focus to be in front of the retina (Fig. 3–1). Thus, the patient's longer-than-normal eye needs more divergent light rays to see. Concave lenses placed in front of the eye diverge the light rays to place the point of focus on the retina (Fig. 3–1).

All ages can have *myopia*: young children who bump into walls, teenagers who fail the school vision test, young adults, and middle-aged adults. It is more common in patients whose parents are myopic.

Patients' Description of Symptoms

Patients may be unable to see signs while driving and/or unable to see distant objects or read the blackboard from the back of the room.

> I can't see the signs on the highway, but everyone else in the car can see them.
>
> I can't see the blackboard.
>
> I can see if I hold the book close to my eyes.

Farsightedness, or Hyperopia

Light rays coming into a short eye cause the point of focus to be behind the eye (Fig. 3–1). Thus, the patient's shorter eye needs to have convergent light rays to see. Convex lenses placed in front of the eye converge the light rays such that the point of focus is placed on the retina (Fig. 3–1).

In young children, the *hyperopia* becomes noticeable because the child may walk into walls. He or she may not be able to focus on nearby objects clearly, or there may be inward crossing of the child's eyes.

Usually, the condition is asymptomatic in young adults until college age, when they spend much time reading and notice headaches with reading.

This entity is common but more asymptomatic than myopia and thus is often unreported.

Patients' Description of Symptoms

> I can't see to read.
>
> I have a headache when I read.
>
> My eyes hurt when I read.

In children, the presentation of a child with "crossed eyes" while reading

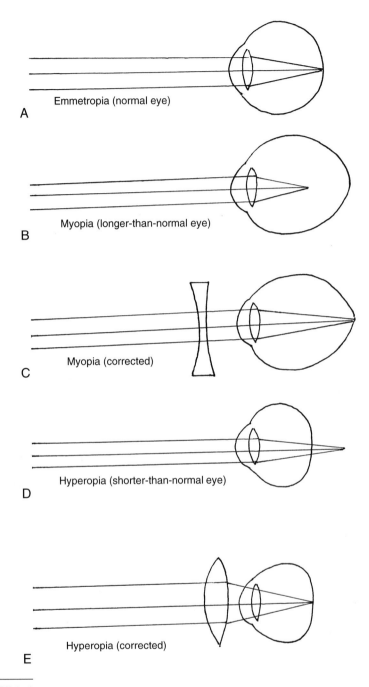

• **FIGURE 3–1**

A, Emmetropia. *B,* Myopia: longer-than-normal eye. *C,* Corrected myopia: concave lens brings the diverging light rays to the retina. *D,* Hyperopia: shorter-than-normal eye. *E,* Corrected hyperopia: convex lens brings the converging light rays to the retina.

also suggests farsightedness. Other children may walk into walls or other near objects.

Presbyopia

The ability to focus at far and near alternately involves the process of accommodation. This phenomenon involves the ability of the lens to change its shape slightly to change the focus of the incoming light rays. This ability decreases as patients approach 40 years of age.

Starting at age 40, patients with presbyopia need to wear reading glasses to aid in the focusing of the light rays for near objects at 16 to 17 inches. The patient's distance vision remains unchanged.

Patients' Description of Symptoms

I can't read the menu at the restaurant.

I can't see the fine print, but I don't need glasses to see in the distance.

Examination

The visual acuity assessment is essential. Using the pinhole improves the tested visual acuity dramatically in some patients. The myope is able to read only the largest letters on the distance Snellen visual acuity chart. The hyperope is able to read only the smallest letters on the distance Snellen visual acuity chart but may have problems with near acuity as tested with the near card. The presbyope is 40 years of age or older and holds the near card as far as his or her arms permit and then reads the card. If the presbyope is tested at the standard 16 inches, he or she is not able to read the near visual acuity card (Table 3–1).

Examination and Management Summary

1. Test with near card and distance Snellen acuity.

2. If pinhole improves vision to 20/20, the patient needs glasses.

TABLE 3–1
EYE EXAMINATION

1. Test the patient's vision with Snellen nearcard and distance Snellen acuity chart.

2. If pinhole device improves vision to 20/20, the patient needs eyeglasses.

3. Send the patient to an ophthalmologist or optometrist for examination and prescription for eyeglasses.

3. Refer to ophthalmologist or optometrist for examination and prescription for glasses.

Eyeglasses

The eye is not harmed if the prescribed glasses are not worn constantly in the adult patient. However, the patient's eyesight is improved by glasses. We recommend that patients leave a pair of eyeglasses in the glove compartments of their cars.

However, children who have been prescribed eyeglasses need to wear them because amblyopia or lazy eye can develop if they do not wear them (see Chapter 9).

Contact Lenses

The wide availability of contact lenses has made this entity popular. However, there has been an accompanying rise in contact lens–related disorders.

SOFT CONTACT LENSES

Soft contact lenses are made up of soft, nonrigid, plastic material that is highly oxygen permeable.

Disposable. These lenses can be everyday disposable or 2-week disposable.

Nondisposable. The life of a contact lens is usually 8 to 12 months. Afterward, protein build-up on lens requires new lens purchase.

Contact Lens Overwear Syndrome
This syndrome is accompanied by pain and poor vision in patients who have had long history of soft contact lens use.

RIGID OR HARD CONTACT LENSES

Rigid or hard contact lenses are made up of hard plastic with varying degrees of oxygen permeability. "Gas-permeable" contact lenses are made up of the most oxygen-permeable material in this class of hard contact lens.

1. Hard contact lenses last for many years or until the curvature of the cornea changes in the patient.

2. These lenses are more prone to corneal abrasions in the novice user.

CARE OF DAILY WEAR CONTACT LENSES AND DISPOSABLE CONTACT LENSES

The care of contact lens must be meticulous, and sterile solutions must be used in the daily cleansing of contact lenses. Otherwise, problems such as corneal abrasions and corneal ulcers can arise. In such cases, once the diagnosis is made, it is best to confer with an ophthalmologist. In the case of a corneal ulcer, in which there is potential for permanent visual loss, referral to an ophthalmologist is necessary for treatment (Table 3–2).

Patients' Description of Symptoms

I can't find my contact lens in my eye, and my eye hurts.

I wore my contact lens to sleep, and I can't open my eye today.

I wore my contact lens for 18 hours, and my eye is red and sore.

Examination

Soft Contact Lens Wearers
1. Examine the patient with a penlight to check the degree of redness.

2. Look to see if there is a contact lens in the eye.

3. Use a drop of proparacaine topical anesthetic eyedrop to relieve patient discomfort.

4. Wear sterile gloves and try to remove the contact lens with your fingers. If that fails, use sterile saline and remove the contact lens by irrigating the eye. Eventually, the lens will slide out.

5. Then, check the eye for a corneal abrasion with the fluorescein strip. If there is no corneal abrasion, consider giving the patient topical ophthalmic antibiotic ointment, such as erythromycin ophthalmic ointment for comfort applied four times a day (QID) for a few days.

Hard Contact Lens Wearers
1. Usually, a hard contact lens is not dislocated, but rather it has caused a scratch on the cornea, causing the patient pain. Use the topical

---

TABLE 3–2

CONTACT LENS USAGE RECOMMENDATIONS

1. All contact lens wearers should see an ophthalmologist regularly.
2. If patient experiences pain while wearing contact lenses, the contact lenses should be removed immediately.
3. Patients should never overwear contact lenses.
4. Patients should follow proper hygiene when using contact lenses.

anesthetic drop proparacaine, and use the fluorescein strip to identify the corneal abrasion.

2. Then, pressure patch the eye: use a drop of the dilating solution 1% cyclopentolate, apply erythromycin ophthalmic ointment, and have the patient close his or her eyes.

3. Then, use two eye patches: fold the first patch over for more bulk, and place it over the upper eyelid; to keep the eye closed, lay the other eye patch on top. Apply both of them diagonally over the closed eyelid.

4. Then, apply tape from the forehead to the zygoma, covering the patch, and repeat until the entire patch is covered (Fig. 3–2).

Examination and Management Summary

1. Use a penlight to examine the eye and assess the situation. Use proparacaine to relieve the patient's discomfort.

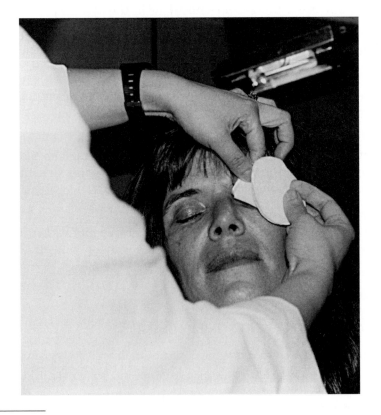

• **FIGURE 3–2**
Pressure patch of the eye. (Photography by Irwin Sterbakov.)

2. If the contact lens is already removed and the eye is still red, use a fluorescein strip to assess the integrity of the cornea.

   a. If the cornea stains green, a corneal abrasion is present. Instill antibiotic ointment (erythromycin ophthalmic ointment) and a dilating drop (1% cyclopentolate), and put two eye patches together and patch the patient's eye shut (Fig. 3–2).

3. If the pain is excruciating, refer the patient to an ophthalmologist immediately. The problem may be unrelated to the contact lens.

4. If a white spot is seen on the cornea, refer the patient to an ophthalmologist immediately. This may be a corneal ulcer.

Pressure Patch Technique for Corneal Abrasion

1. Instill proparacaine eyedrops.

2. Instill 1% cyclopentolate eyedrops.

3. Use two eye patches: fold the first over, for more bulk, and place it over the upper eyelid; to keep the eye closed, lay the other eye patch on top. Apply both of them diagonally over the closed eyelid.

4. Apply tape from the forehead to the zygoma, covering the patch, and repeat until the entire eye patch is covered (Fig. 3–2).

SKIN AND ADNEXAL DISORDERS

Infections

CHALAZION AND HORDEOLUM

The inspissation of the meibomian glands, the small glands that accompany each cilium on the eyelids, causes an erythematous discoloration on the eyelid. These glands are sandwiched between the tarsus, the underside of the eyelid, and the epidermal layer of the eyelid. Because very little potential space exists, any swelling is felt acutely by the patient. After 1 to 2 weeks, edema, irritation, and pain may be present (Fig. 3–3; see also Fig. 3–3 Color Plate 1). Occasionally, a white cheesy discharge may emanate from the orifices of the meibomian glands (see Chapter 1, Table 1–1). At the 2- to 4-week stage, the swollen area in the eyelid hardens, and it becomes chronically indurated. At the chronic stage, this is a granulomatous infection and is called a *chalazion*. In the acute stage, when there is much edema and erythema and pain, it is called a *hordeolum*.

This condition is common in childhood and adolescence. Women who use heavy eye make-up also tend to have this condition. It is more common on

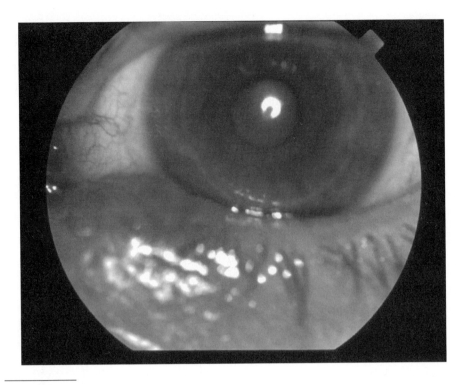

• **FIGURE 3–3**
Chalazion.

the upper eyelids. It can occur in each eye and on upper and lower eyelids simultaneously. It is usually caused by the staphylococcal family of bacteria.

Patients' Description of Symptoms

I have a stye.

I have had pain over my eyelid for a month, and now I have a lump.

My eyelid is swollen shut.

Examination and Management Summary

1. Examine the eye by simple inspection. Instruct the patient to look downward. Pull gently on the upper eyelid to view the underside of the eyelid to identify any localized edema or masses.

2. Examine the other eye in a similar fashion.

3. For treatment of the chalazion, apply warm compresses with a clean face towel or paper towel to dissipate some of the swelling.

TABLE 3–3
CHALAZION MANAGEMENT

1. Apply warm compresses four times a day.
2. Apply erythromycin ophthalmic ointment afterward.

4. Apply warm compresses four times a day, and apply erythromycin ophthalmic ointment four times a day to the affected eye. Erythromycin ophthalmic ointment is not irritating to the cornea. For patients allergic to erythromycin, bacitracin ophthalmic ointment is a good substitute (Table 3–3).

5. For chronic infections of at least 4 weeks' duration, refer the patient to an ophthalmologist for further evaluation and treatment. The ophthalmologist can perform excisional surgery at his or her office.

PRESEPTAL CELLULITIS

When the hordeolum or chalazion progresses in patients with poor hygiene or in diabetic patients, the edema and erythema spread to the upper and lower eyelids (Fig. 3–4; see also Fig. 3–4 Color Plate 1). This condition is

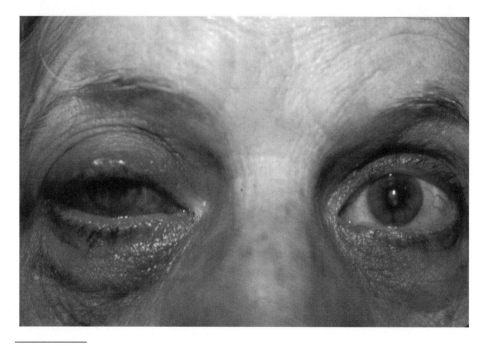

• **FIGURE 3–4**
Preseptal cellulitis.

TABLE 3–4
PRESEPTAL CELLULITIS MANAGEMENT

1. Administer oral antibiotics: penicillin VK, 500 mg QID PO for 10 days.

2. If no improvement is seen after 1 week, refer the patient to an ophthalmologist.

QID = four times a day; PO = by mouth.

called *preseptal cellulitis*. The treatment for preseptal cellulitis is oral antibiotics for gram-positive coverage, such as penicillin VK 500 mg by mouth QID
for 10 days (Table 3–4).

ORBITAL CELLULITIS

When the infection extends to the orbital rim and deeper tissues, it is
called *orbital cellulitis*. The patient is usually febrile and experiences malaise
and visual loss. Severe pain and headache may be present. At this point,
unilateral involvement of the eyelids and the orbital region is present (Fig.
3–5; see also Fig. 3–5 Color Plate 1).

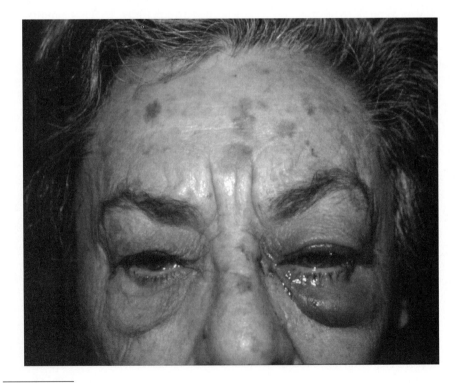

• **FIGURE 3–5**
Orbital cellulitis.

The organisms responsible for the infection are usually streptococci or staphylococci, the same organisms responsible for acute sinusitis involving the ethmoidal, sphenoidal, maxillary, or frontal sinuses.

In children, orbital cellulitis can occur in association with sinusitis because of the contiguous location of the sinus cells and the orbit. Bacterial invasion can occur through vascular channels or through direct extension through the orbit and the sinuses.

The ophthalmologist should be consulted at the beginning of treatment so that the primary care physician and ophthalmologist can coordinate the care of the patient. The treatment at this point is intravenous antibiotics. If after 2 to 3 days of antibiotic therapy the patient does not seem to get better, surgical drainage should be considered by the ophthalmologist (Table 3–5).

Examination and Management Summary

1. Examine the patient with a penlight to determine the extent of the erythema.

2. Check the pupils.

3. If the redness extends to upper and lower eyelids, without involvement of the pupil, give oral antibiotics.

4. If the pupillary response to light is abnormal and associated with pain or visual loss, consider the patient's condition to be more serious, and refer the patient to an ophthalmologist immediately.

5. If the pupillary response is not clear but the patient has severe pain, visual loss, and fever, refer the patient to an ophthalmologist immediately.

DACRYOCYSTITIS

Dacryocystitis occurs in the elderly population. The lacrimal system in the elderly becomes obstructed, and poor drainage causes a pus-filled abscess

---

TABLE 3–5

ORBITAL CELLULITIS

1. Examine eye with penlight.
2. Check pupils.
3. If the redness extends to upper and lower eyelids, without involvement of the pupil, give oral antibiotics.
4. If an abnormal pupillary response is associated with pain or visual loss, refer to an ophthalmologist immediately.

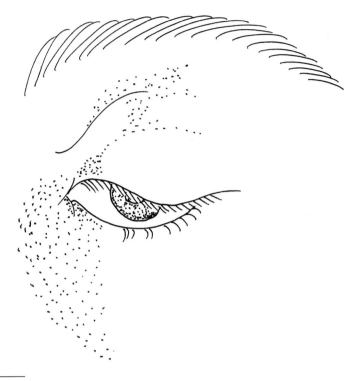

• **FIGURE 3–6**
Swelling at the medial canthus, dacryocystitis.

cavity within the lacrimal system. There is an outpouching of an abscess-like sac at the medial canthus associated with pain, edema, and erythema (Fig. 3–6). There is active purulent secretion. The eye seems to be displaced laterally. The most likely pathogen is *Staphylococcus aureus.* Less commonly, other organisms, such as *Actinomyces,* in immunocompromised hosts, can be responsible (Table 3–6).

Surgical drainage is usually necessary in severe cases. However, antibiotics are used to pretreat the infection before surgery. Gram-positive coverage is necessary. Culture and sensitivity of the purulent secretion provide guide-

TABLE 3–6
DACRYOCYSTITIS

1. Look at the medial canthal area of the eye. If a mass is present, gently palpate it and observe if purulence is released.

2. Culture the purulent material.

3. Start oral antibiotic therapy.

4. Refer the patient to an ophthalmologist if there is no improvement.

lines for antibiotic treatment. Consultation with an ophthalmologist is advised at this point.

Examination and Management Summary

1. Look at the medial canthal area of the eye. If a mass is present, gently palpate it and observe if purulence is released.

2. Culture the purulent material.

3. Begin oral antibiotic therapy.

Inflammation

GRAVES' DISEASE

Graves' disease is an autoimmune process that leads to infiltration by large numbers of chronic inflammatory cells, deposition of mucopolysaccharides, and increased extracellular volume. This disease can occur in patients with hyperthyroidism. However, patients may manifest ophthalmic signs of Graves' disease without clinical evidence of hyperthyroidism. These patients are considered to have ophthalmic Graves' disease.

Patients may have nonspecific complaints of dryness or foreign body sensation of the eyes. Usually, if the symptoms abate after treatment of artificial tears, no further work-up is needed. If dryness persists after months of treatment, laboratory evaluation of thyroid dysfunction should be considered. In chronic ophthalmic Graves' disease, periorbital edema, red eyes, conjunctival edema (chemosis), and proptosis occur (Figs. 3–7 and 3–8; see also Fig. 3–7 Color Plate 1). Computed tomography can demonstrate the swelling of the extraocular muscles; this phenomenon accounts for the proptosis. Complications include corneal exposure and optic neuropathy resulting from compression of the optic nerve by enlarged extraocular muscles at the apex of the orbital cone. Treatment at this stage consists of high doses of systemic steroids and surgical decompression of the orbit. The American Thyroid Association has graded the ocular signs by class (Table 3–7).

Examination and Management Summary

1. Observe the proptosis from the profile view of the face and observe the facial asymmetry at the eye and orbital region.

2. Instruct the patient to close his or her eyes. Then, gently palpate the area around the orbit for fullness.

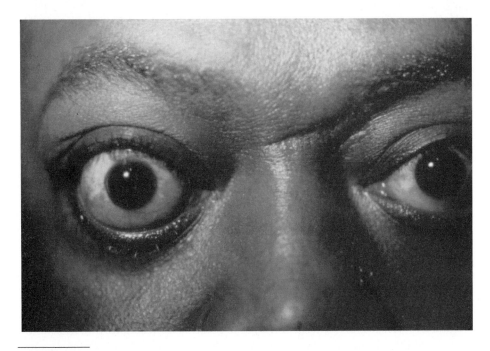

• **FIGURE 3–7**
Graves' disease with unequal edema of the eyelids.

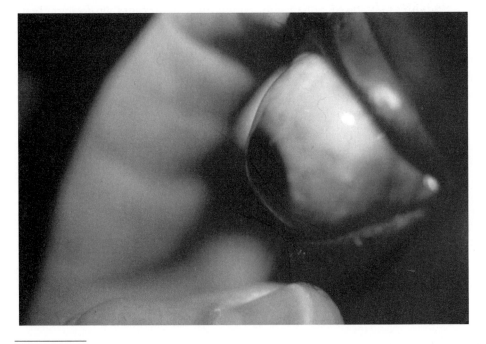

• **FIGURE 3–8**
Graves' disease with proptosis.

TABLE 3–7

AMERICAN THYROID ASSOCIATION OCULAR SIGNS

Class	Signs
0	No signs or symptoms
1	Only signs, upper eyelid retraction, with or without eyelid lag or proptosis, no symptoms
2	Soft tissue involvement
3	Proptosis
4	Extraocular muscle involvement
5	Corneal involvement
6	Sight loss due to optic nerve involvement

3. Evaluate the pupils and the extraocular movements because there may be restriction of gaze or obvious asymmetry when the patient gazes rightward, leftward, upward, and downward.

4. Refer the patient to an ophthalmologist if the patient complains of eye symptoms despite treatment with artificial tears. At that point, surgical decompression of the eyelid and optic nerve may be necessary at the hands of the ophthalmic surgeon.

5. Treatment involves control of the primary thyroid disease. In severe cases of visual loss, management of the patient may be necessary with the ophthalmologist and primary care physician.

6. For class 0 to 2 involvement (see Table 3–7: no signs or symptoms, or upper eyelid retraction, eyelid lag, asymptomatic proptosis, and soft tissue involvement), treatment is directed at patient comfort, that is, use of artificial tears as often as necessary (QID to once an hour while awake) and use of artificial tear lubricant at night.

7. For class 3 to 5 involvement (see Table 3–7: proptosis, extraocular muscle involvement, corneal involvement), consultation with an ophthalmic surgeon is indicated.

8. For class 6 involvement (see Table 3–7: visual loss due to optic nerve involvement), immediate consultation with an ophthalmic surgeon is indicated.

Eyelid Disorders

ENTROPION

Entropion is the inversion of the eyelid, causing the inwardly turned eyelashes to brush against the cornea. It usually affects the lower eyelid more than the upper eyelid (Fig. 3–9). In the elderly, it is called *senile entropion*,

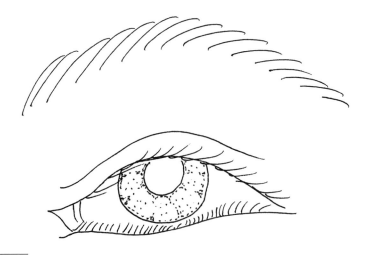

• **FIGURE 3–9**
Entropion.

caused by the degeneration of the fascial attachments in the lower eyelid and dehiscence of the lower eyelid retractors from the lower eyelid tarsus.

Cicatricial entropion is caused by scarring of the palpebral conjunctiva and the tarsus. This can happen in a younger age group and can be caused by trachoma or trauma to the eye.

Usually, the patient complains of irritation of the eyelids, and, over time, the patient may have decreased vision in the affected eye (Table 3–8).

Examination and Management Summary

1. Examination reveals an inverted lower eyelid with the eyelashes rubbing against the cornea on blinking.

2. The management in severe cases is surgery to evert the eyelid.

3. In mild cases or in infirm patients in nursing homes, the lower eyelid can be taped to the cheek with tension temporally and inferiorly; this measure may alleviate the problem.

TABLE 3–8
ECTROPION AND ENTROPION MANAGEMENT

1. Prescribe artificial tears (eyedrop or ointment form).
2. If the patient has deteriorating vision, refer him or her to an ophthalmologist.

4. Artificial tear lubricant ointments and artificial tear replacements are useful as well.

ECTROPION

Ectropion is the sagging and consequent eversion of the lower eyelid, usually bilateral (Fig. 3–10). It is common in the elderly population. Ectropion may be caused by the relaxation of the orbicularis oculi muscle, as part of the aging process or seventh nerve palsy. The symptoms are tearing and irritation. The cornea may become severely dry and cause a temporary decrease in vision.

Examination and Management Summary

1. Penlight examination reveals the eversion of the lower eyelid and the poor apposition of the lower eyelid against the cornea.

2. Treatment consists of replacement tears and tear ointment. Surgery is recommended for severe cases.

PTOSIS

Ptosis is the bilateral or unilateral drooping of the upper eyelid (Fig. 3–11). It can be congenital, resulting from developmental failure of the levator

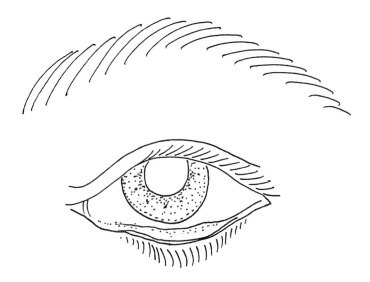

• **FIGURE 3–10**
Ectropion.

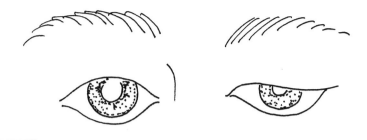

• **FIGURE 3–11**
Ptosis.

muscle of the eyelid, alone or in association with anomalies of the superior rectus muscle. This condition can be present at birth or shortly after birth.

Acquired ptosis can be due to swelling, tumor, or chronic inflammation. Ptosis of both eyelids may be due to myogenic factors, such as myasthenia gravis and muscular dystrophy. In myasthenia gravis, the defect is in the humoral transmission at the myoneural junction.

Neurogenic or paralytic ptosis is due to a third nerve palsy from central nervous system problems or cerebrovascular accidents.

Examination and Management

Examination reveals an inability to raise the eyelid. The deformity may be so slight that no correction is necessary. In cases of congenital ptosis in children, the ptotic eyelid obscures the pupil, preventing normal visual development; surgery should be performed to prevent amblyopia or lazy eye. Surgical evaluation can be deferred to an ophthalmologist (Table 3–8).

Examination and Management Summary

1. Look with penlight to ascertain the eyelid deformity.

2. If the eyelid is inverted, try using tape to evert it gently. Use of artificial tear lubricants is helpful if the condition is not severe. Otherwise, a referral to an ophthalmologist for eyelid surgery is advised.

3. If the eyelid is inverted, tear lubrication may not solve the long-term problem. The patient requires eyelid surgery with an ophthalmologist.

4. If the eyelid is covering part of the eye asymmetrically and the adult patient cannot see, then referral to an ophthalmologist is necessary. If the ptosis is mild and causes no concern in the adult patient, referral is not needed.

5. Children with ptosis need to be referred to an ophthalmologist for evaluation because they may have other structural abnormalities and may require glasses.

Benign Tumors

MILIA

Milia are small, white, benign cystic lesions, measuring 1 mm, near the eyelids. They are not surrounded by any signs of inflammation (Fig. 3–12). These small lesions are bothersome to the patient for cosmetic reasons. They can occur in the second and third decades of life. Excision should be performed by the ophthalmologist, for cosmetic reasons only.

PAPILLOMA

Papillomas are benign, lightly pigmented lesions around the eyelids, with furrows, at the eyelid margins. They can grow larger over the period of several years. The rate of growth is very slow (Fig. 3–12). They are sometimes cosmetically bothersome to the patient. Treatment, if any, is excisional biopsy by the ophthalmologist.

KERATOACANTHOMA

Keratoacanthomas have a pearly center with raised margins (Fig. 3–13). They can mimic basal cell carcinoma, especially in the elderly, and can

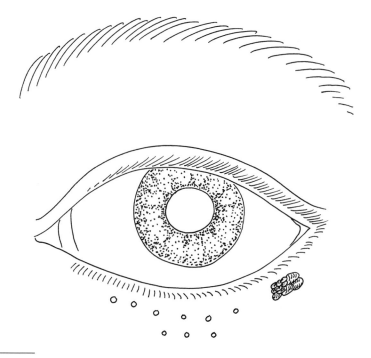

• **FIGURE 3–12**
Milia *(lesion on the left);* papilloma *(lesion on the right).*

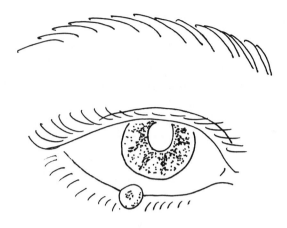

• **FIGURE 3–13**
Keratoacanthoma.

manifest with ulcerated margins if the patient has a history of chronically poor eyelid hygiene. However, they are benign. Keratoacanthomas are common in the elderly in the sixth, seventh, and eighth decades of life.

NEVUS

Nevi are pigmented flat lesions around the eyelids and orbit. Sometimes, hair arises from a nevus. These lesions need to be photographed and observed annually. The patient should be warned about color change or size change. No treatment is necessary (Fig. 3–14).

Iris nevi are unilateral or bilateral darkly pigmented lesions of the iris. Patients with these lesions should be referred to an ophthalmologist for further evaluation of the retina and internal structures of the eye. The lesions can be associated with malignant lesions inside the eye, seen only by ophthalmoscopy with dilating eyedrops (Fig. 3–15; see also Fig. 3–15 Color Plate 1).

XANTHELASMA

Xanthelasmas are benign, oval, yellow plaques measuring 4 to 7 mm distributed around the upper and lower eyelids, usually bilaterally (Fig. 3–16; see also Fig. 3–16 Color Plate 2). They can be found along the lower orbital rim bilaterally as well. They are slightly raised and uniform in color. They are caused by cholesterol deposits around the skin. Usually, the patient has accompanying elevated cholesterol levels. Unfortunately, with the medical treatment of hypercholesterolemia, these xanthelasmas do not resolve. Usually, no treatment is necessary, and if cosmetic surgery is desired, an ophthalmologist can perform the outpatient surgery to remove the lesions.

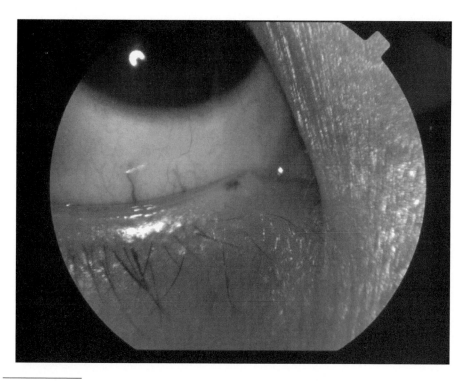

• **FIGURE 3–14**
Nevus at the medial canthal region.

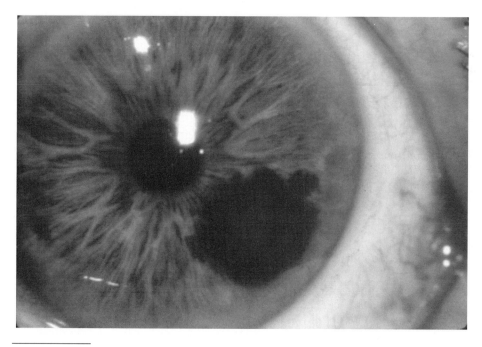

• **FIGURE 3–15**
Iris nevus.

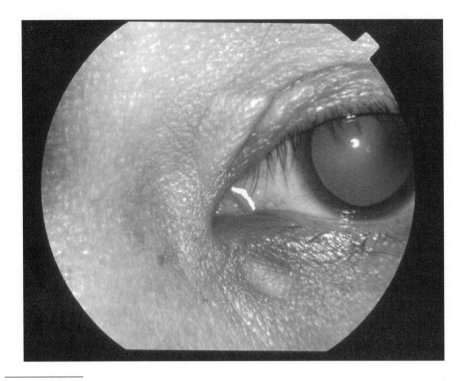

• **FIGURE 3–16**
Xanthelasma.

DERMOID

Dermoids are lesions found under the eyelids or at the edge of the medial canthus in children. They are smooth, encapsulated, and avascular (Fig. 3–17). These lesions may be accompanied by other developmental anomalies of the eyeball, and patients with them should be referred to an ophthalmologist for further evaluation. The ophthalmologist examines the patient for orbital involvement with ophthalmic ultrasonography or computed tomography. In addition, the patient is examined for any anomalies of the retina.

Examination and Management Summary

1. Inspect and look for any erythema, induration, abnormal vascularity, or coloration. The benign lesions are in the setting of normal skin coloration and do not disturb the anatomy of the eye.

2. If the lesion is questionable, ask for ophthalmic consultation.

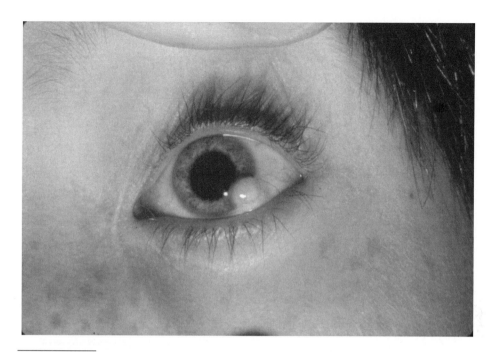

• **FIGURE 3–17**
Dermoid.

Malignant Tumors

BASAL CELL CARCINOMA

Basal cell carcinoma is a common eyelid lesion on sun-exposed areas of the face. The physician should look for nonhealing ulcerated lesions. These lesions can be small, measuring 3 to 10 mm. They can be overlooked by the patient. They are common around the eyelids and on the nose (Fig. 3–18; see also Fig. 3–18 Color Plate 2). Patients with these lesions need to be referred to a dermatologist or an ophthalmologist for an evaluation and possible excisional biopsy.

SQUAMOUS CELL CARCINOMA

These lesions are ulcerating and have areas of eschar formation (Fig. 3–19; see also Fig. 3–19 Color Plate 2). They tend to be present in a more dramatic manner than basal cell carcinomas and are more aggressive. Patients with these lesions need immediate referral to an ophthalmologist.

LYMPHOMA

These lesions are infiltrative and present as a salmon-colored mass lesion near the medial canthus or lateral canthus (Fig. 3–20; see also Fig. 3–20

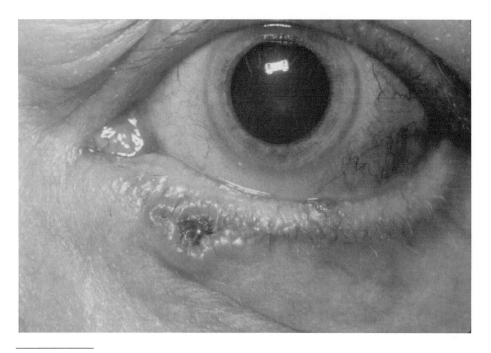

• **FIGURE 3–18**
Basal cell carcinoma. (Courtesy of Peter Rubin, MD, Boston, MA.)

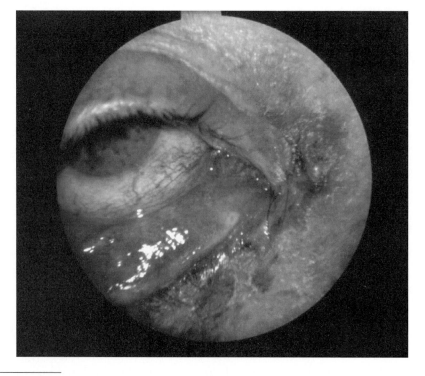

• **FIGURE 3–19**
Squamous cell carcinoma.

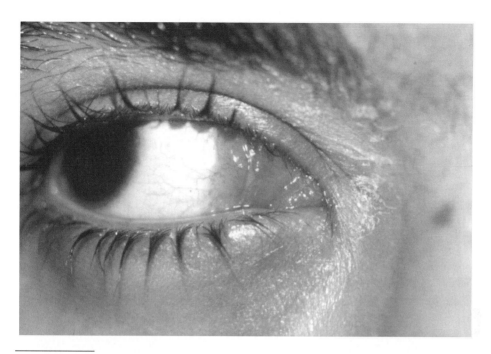

• **FIGURE 3–20**
Lymphoma of the medial canthus.

Color Plate 2). On eversion of the upper or lower eyelids, these lesions may extend to surround part of the eye. These need further evaluation with diagnostic ultrasonography, computed tomography, or magnetic resonance imaging of the orbit to delineate their extension. A diagnostic work-up for the underlying malignancy is usually initiated at the primary care physician's office. Then, the patient is usually referred to an ophthalmologist specializing in tumors for surgical treatment or radiation treatment if the tumor is extensive.

MALIGNANT MELANOMA

Intraocular *malignant melanoma* occurs in an estimated six cases per one million people per year. It is the most common intraocular malignancy of the Caucasian population. The average age of diagnosis is the sixth decade. The tumor is seen in its early stages during routine ophthalmologic evaluations in asymptomatic patients or in patients presenting with blurred vision. Glaucoma may be a late manifestation.

The patient may not have symptoms unless the tumor affects the line of sight (Fig. 3–21; see also Fig. 3–21 Color Plate 2). In late stages, the tumor size may be large, thus causing a retinal detachment with concomitant loss of vision. The tumor may be located in the iris and may change the color of the iris or deform the pupil.

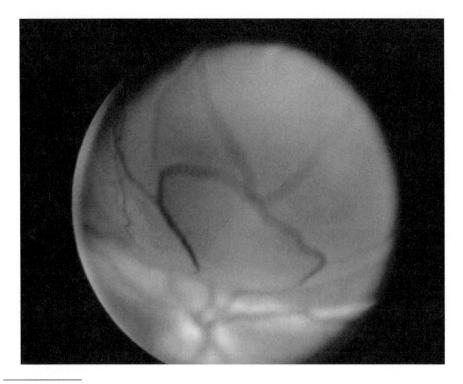

• **FIGURE 3–21**
Malignant melanoma.

Management
    The patient should be referred to an ophthalmologist for diagnosis. After the diagnosis is made, an oncologic evaluation is coordinated by the primary care physician, ophthalmologist, and radiologist.

Treatment
    Enucleation of the blind eye has been the traditional treatment. Other modes of therapy, such as radiotherapy with cobalt plaques and charged-particle irradiation, may be used. Laser therapy and cryotherapy have been used with small tumors.

Examination and Management Summary

1. Look with the penlight to observe any observable masses in the iris, or, with the direct ophthalmoscope, observe any discolored masses inside the retina.

2. Refer the patient to an ophthalmologist if there is any question of mass lesion.

CONJUNCTIVAL DISORDERS

Conjunctivitis

VIRAL CONJUNCTIVITIS

Most cases of conjunctivitis are caused by viruses. *Viral conjunctivitis* presents as a bilateral but asymmetric swelling of the eyelids and injection of the conjunctivae; viral conjunctivitis may or may not be associated with upper respiratory tract infection. Usually, there is associated preauricular lymph node swelling in the course of the process. Viral conjunctivitis is self-limited, but the treatment is directed toward symptomatic relief, that is, foreign body sensation or tearing (Fig. 3–22).

In severe viral infections, which can last for up to 6 months, the symptoms are usually severe injection of the conjunctivae with decreased vision. In these cases, a referral to an ophthalmologist may be necessary (Table 3–9 and Fig. 3–22).

HERPES SIMPLEX CONJUNCTIVITIS

Herpetic conjunctivitis may present as mucocutaneous ulceration of the eyelid margin. The conjunctiva is ulcerated on eversion. In addition, small ulcerated skin lesions may occur that form crusting during the first week of the infection. Herpetic conjunctivitis is associated with large preauricular lymph nodes. Corneal involvement can occur, and the patient should be referred to an ophthalmologist for further treatment (Table 3–9).

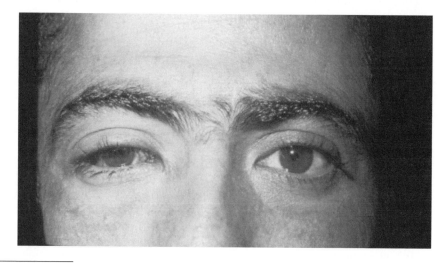

• **FIGURE 3–22**
Viral conjunctivitis.

TABLE 3–9

CONJUNCTIVITIS MANAGEMENT

1. Use gloves when examining patients with conjunctivitis to prevent spread of the virus to other patients.

2. If patient has clear discharge associated with upper respiratory infection, consider a diagnosis of viral conjunctivitis. Antibiotic therapy is not necessary, but to prevent bacterial superinfection, apply erythromycin ophthalmic ointment QID to the affected eye.

3. If purulent discharge is present, culture the discharge and start appropriate antibiotic therapy in ointment form.

4. If herpesvirus infection is suspected, look for skin vesicles or herpes zoster–like skin lesions. Refer patients with this condition to an ophthalmologist for further evaluation and treatment.

QID = four times a day.

Management

Treatment consists of administration of trifluridine eyedrops five to 10 times a day.

HERPES ZOSTER CONJUNCTIVITIS AND KERATITIS

In this condition, the patient has the usual vesicular skin lesions in the distribution of the trigeminal nerve. If there is involvement of the tip of the nose, then likelihood that the cornea will be involved as well is greater (Fig. 3–23; see also Fig. 3–23 Color Plate 2). Patients with this condition need to be referred to an ophthalmologist (see Table 3–9 and Fig. 3–22).

Management

Corticosteroid drops and oral acyclovir treatment are helpful.

Examination and Management Summary

1. Use gloves when examining patients with conjunctivitis to prevent spread of the virus to other patients.

2. If clear discharge associated with upper respiratory infection is present, consider a diagnosis of viral conjunctivitis. Antibiotic therapy is unnecessary, but to prevent bacterial superinfection, erythromycin ophthalmic ointment should be applied QID to the affected eye.

3. If you suspect herpesvirus infection, look for skin vesicles or herpes zoster–like skin lesions. Refer these patients to an ophthalmologist for further evaluation and treatment.

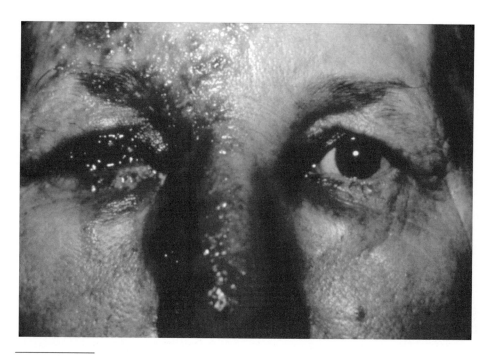

• **FIGURE 3–23**
Herpes zoster conjunctivitis.

BACTERIAL CONJUNCTIVITIS

Acute onset and profuse, thick, purulent discharge characterize bacterial conjunctivitis (Fig. 3–24; see also Fig. 3–24 Color Plate 3). There usually is a rapid response to topical antibiotics. Culture of the conjunctiva is helpful in chronic cases. The most common causative organisms are *Staphylococcus, Pneumococcus, Moraxella, Hemophilus*, and gonococcus (see Table 3–9 and Fig. 3–23; see also Fig. 3–23 Color Plate 2).

Examination and Management Summary

1. If the discharge is thick and purulent, consider a diagnosis of bacterial conjunctivitis.

2. Culture the purulent discharge.

3. Erythromycin ophthalmic or bacitracin ophthalmic ointment can be applied QID to the affected eye.

Nevus

Conjunctival nevus is hyperpigmentation in an irregular pattern of the conjunctiva (Fig. 3–25). It can be present at birth. New pigmentation can

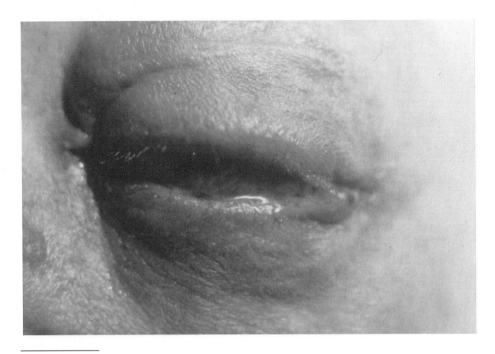

• **FIGURE 3–24**
Gonorrheal conjunctivitis with purulence.

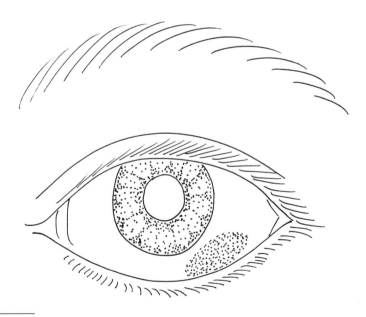

• **FIGURE 3–25**
Conjunctival nevus.

arise in the fourth decade of life. It is important to monitor the growth or any pigment changes of these lesions because they do have a malignant potential. These new areas of pigmentation are called *acquired melanosis*.

Acquired melanosis in Caucasian individuals is significant because it may represent a premalignant condition. The physician can document this condition with drawings, noting the size, extent, and coloration at presentation.

Conjunctival Tumors

PAPILLOMA

Papilloma are pink, pedunculated lesions with an irregular surface, occurring at the medial canthal region or at the lateral canthus. Occasionally, the lesions are multiple. If the papilloma arises at the limbus, it may invade the cornea. Treatment is excisional biopsy by an ophthalmologist.

BOWEN'S DISEASE OR CARCINOMA IN SITU OF THE CONJUNCTIVA

These diseases appear as elevated, vascular reddish-gray mass lesions associated with an inflammatory reaction. Treatment is excisional biopsy by an ophthalmologist.

SQUAMOUS CELL CARCINOMA OF THE CONJUNCTIVA

Squamous cell carcinoma presents as a rare, limbal, small gray nodule extending into the cornea and around the adjacent areas of the conjunctiva. Treatment is excisional biopsy. If the invasion is extensive, further diagnostic testing may be needed at an ophthalmologist's office.

HEMANGIOMA OF THE CONJUNCTIVA

Hemangioma is a lesion with a reddish coloration that presents for many years without changes. No treatment is needed.

MALIGNANT MELANOMA OF THE CONJUNCTIVA

This tumor arises spontaneously from an existing nevus or an area of precancerous melanosis (Fig. 3–25). Males and females are equally affected. It occurs between the ages of 40 and 60 years. Excisional biopsy and/or cryosurgery by the ophthalmologist is necessary (Fig. 3–26; see also Fig. 3–26 Color Plate 3).

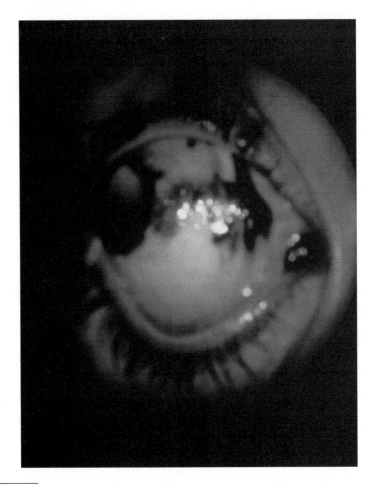

• **FIGURE 3–26**
Conjunctival melanoma.

Examination and Management Summary

1. Inspect for abnormalities in size, coloration, or growth pattern.

2. If a lesion is questionable, ask for an ophthalmic consultation.

DISEASES OF THE CORNEA

Superficial Trauma to the Cornea: Corneal Abrasion

A corneal abrasion is a scratch on the clear part of the eye. It can be caused by an accidental flick of the fingernail, a paper cut to the eye, or a child's playful swipe at the cornea (Fig. 3–27). It usually heals within 24 to

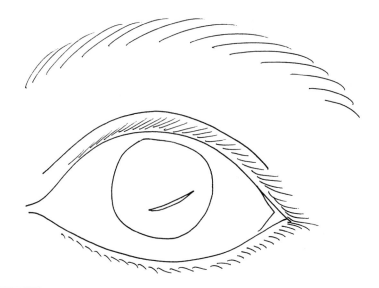

• **FIGURE 3–27**
Corneal abrasion.

48 hours, with cycloplegic drops, antibiotic ointment, and pressure patching
(Fig. 3–2) (see Contact Lenses section).

Keratitis

BACTERIAL KERATITIS

Once superficial trauma occurs to the cornea, invasion of local organisms
can occur. The most likely pathogens are those in the staphylococcal family.
In contact lens wearers, other pathogens also include *Streptococcus, Pseudo-
monas, Klebsiella,* and *Moraxella*. Characteristic of *bacterial keratitis* is pain,
decreased vision, hyperemia of the conjunctiva, and purulent discharge. Culture and sensitivities are important for identification of the organism. Patients with this condition should be referred to an ophthalmologist.

FUNGAL KERATITIS

In agricultural settings where plant and vegetable matter is abundant, a
foreign body in the cornea can lead to an indolent *fungal infection*. Symptoms
may arise weeks and months later. The cornea may present with a gray
infiltrate, hypopyon, marked injection, and superficial ulceration (Fig. 3–28).
The most common fungal organisms are *Candida, Fusarium, Aspergillus*, and
Penicillium.

Patients with this condition should be referred to an ophthalmologist for

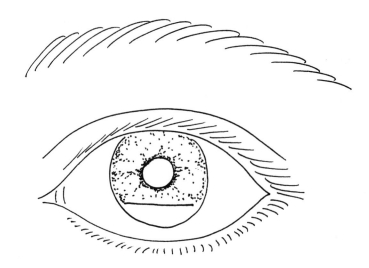

• **FIGURE 3–28**
Hypopyon in fungal keratitis.

scrapings of the corneal ulcer. The specimens should be sent to an infectious disease laboratory for identification, culture, and sensitivity.

VIRAL KERATITIS

Herpes simplex keratitis is the ocular counterpart of oral herpes. The associated fever blister is present near the eyelids in young infants and young adults. In the cornea, using fluorescein and a flashlight with a blue filter, the primary care physician can sometimes see a dendrite (Fig. 3–29; see also Fig. 3–29 Color Plate 3).

The symptoms are irritation, photophobia, and tearing. When the central cornea is affected, decreased vision occurs.

Recurrent herpes simplex keratitis is triggered by fever, overexposure to ultraviolet light, trauma, psychic stress, onset of menstruation, or some local or systemic source of immunosuppression. It is usually unilateral but can be bilateral.

Treatment consists of administration of trifluridine eyedrops. However, the patient should be referred to an ophthalmologist for examination and further management. The ophthalmologist has specialized equipment, such as the slit-lamp biomicroscope, which allows for careful follow-up.

Corneal Ulcers

Keratitis can develop into *corneal ulcers* when there is colonization of the cornea by the offending pathogenic organism. The patient must be referred

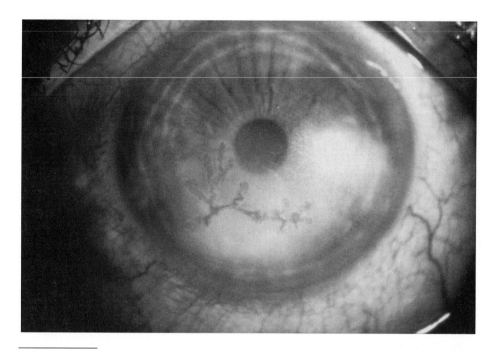

• **FIGURE 3–29**
Dendrite in herpes simplex keratitis. (From American Academy of Ophthalmology. External Disease and Cornea: A Multimedia Collection. San Francisco: American Academy of Ophthalmology, 1994.)

to an ophthalmologist for immediate treatment and sometimes systemic and hourly corneal eyedrops. In some cases, hospitalization may be necessary (Table 3–10).

Examination and Management Summary

1. Using a penlight, identify any white lesions on the cornea, note erythema of the eyelid, and redness of the conjunctiva.

2. Note purulent discharge.

3. Immediately refer the patient to an ophthalmologist for evaluation

---

TABLE 3–10
KERATITIS MANAGEMENT

1. Use a penlight to identify any white lesions on the cornea.

2. Note purulent discharge.

3. Immediately refer the patient to an ophthalmologist for evaluation and management.

and management. Occasionally, this presentation of corneal keratitis and corneal ulcer may require immediate hospitalization and surgery by an ophthalmologist.

Dry Eye and Associated Systemic Disease

Tears are a mixture of secretions from the lacrimal glands, goblet cells of the conjunctiva, and meibomian glands (see Chapter 1). Tears are composed of three layers: (1) a superficial lipid layer from the meibomian glands; (2) a water-soluble, aqueous layer made up of salts and proteins from the lacrimal glands; and (3) a mucinous, hydrophobic layer elaborated by the goblet cells of the conjunctiva. In the syndrome of *dry eye*, a deficiency of any or all three of these tear film layers occurs.

Patients have a foreign body or "sandy" sensation of the eyes. However, in most patients, the eye examination is grossly normal.

Conditions Associated with Dry Eye

HYPOFUNCTION OF THE LACRIMAL GLAND

Hypofunction of the lacrimal gland may occur in Sjögren's syndrome; systemic disease with lacrimal gland involvement, such as sarcoid, lymphoma, leukemia, amyloidosis, and hemochromatosis; drug effects of atropine, diuretics, general anesthetics, and beta-adrenergic blockers, such as atenolol, metoprolol, propranolol, acebutolol, pindolol, and timolol; trachoma; surgical removal of the lacrimal gland; mumps; and old age.

EXCESSIVE EVAPORATION OF TEARS

Excessive evaporation of tears can be caused by exposure keratitis caused by seventh nerve palsy, neuroparalytic keratitis; dry climate, such as desert areas; deficiency of the superficial lipid layer; eyelid surgery; eyelid deformities; and ectropion.

MUCIN DEFICIENCY

Mucin deficiency can be caused by avitaminosis A; Stevens-Johnson syndrome; pemphigoid; trachoma; chemical burns; chronic bacterial or viral conjunctivitis; and drugs, such as antihistamines and anticholinergic agents.

Treatment

Treatment consists of use of artificial tears and artificial tear ointment. In chronic dry eye, evaluation of an underlying systemic disorder can be undertaken as well (Table 3–11).

TABLE 3–11
DRY EYE MANAGEMENT

1. If the patient has discomfort, use artificial tears or ointment.
2. If the problem is chronic, try a trial of artificial tear replacement.
3. If the problem is acute, try to find an environmental cause for the discomfort.
4. If questions persist, refer the patient to an ophthalmologist.

Examination and Management Summary

1. Obtain a good history: does the patient have discomfort?

2. If the problem is chronic, try a trial of artificial tear replacement.

3. If the problem is acute, try to find out an environmental cause for the discomfort.

4. If questions persist, obtain an ophthalmic referral. The ophthalmologist would be able to see certain conditions with the slit-lamp biomicroscope.

ABNORMALITIES OF THE PUPIL

Unequal Pupils

The size of the normal pupil varies between 3 and 4 mm; it is larger in childhood and progressively smaller with advancing age. Myopic patients have larger pupils. Patients using pilocarpine eyedrops have very small pupils. Many normal patients have a slight difference in pupil size of l mm.

Afferent Pupillary Defect

A relative *afferent pupillary defect* is an objective sign of an asymmetric lesion of the afferent visual system (retina, optic nerve, chiasm, or optic tract carrying the pupillary fibers).

The examination of an afferent pupillary defect consists of stimulation of one eye by a bright flashlight, producing an equal constricting response in both eyes as a result of the direct and consensual light reflexes. If the afferent visual system is normal, transfer of the light to the fellow eye maintains the same constriction and tone on both pupils. If an asymmetric lesion exists in the afferent visual pathways, the transfer of the light from the good eye to the bad eye results in less stimulation of the Edinger-Westphal nucleus from that eye and a comparative dilation of both pupils (Figs. 3–30 to 3–33; Table 3–12).

Adie's Pupil

In some patients, a small difference (1 mm) may exist in the pupil size, which may be noticeable to patients because of increased sensitivity to light. A weak 1/8% solution of pilocarpine instilled into the conjunctival sac causes the atonic pupil to constrict, whereas the normal pupil is not affected. The tonic pupil dilates slowly in the dark and reacts promptly to mydriatics.

Adie's pupil is caused by a lesion of the ciliary ganglion. With time, deep tendon reflexes can be lost. Sector iris atrophy can be seen as well.

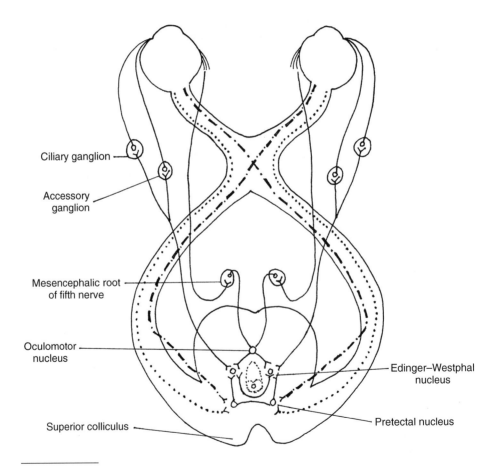

Ciliary ganglion

Accessory ganglion

Mesencephalic root of fifth nerve

Oculomotor nucleus

Edinger–Westphal nucleus

Pretectal nucleus

Superior colliculus

• **FIGURE 3–30**
Pathway of pupillary light reflex.

TABLE 3–12
PUPILLARY EXAMINATION

1. Perform the test for pupillary reaction at near and distance.

2. Is there a relative afferent pupillary response? (This response may result from an asymmetric lesion of the afferent visual system.)

3. Adie's pupil shows a 1-mm difference between both pupils.

4. Refer the patient to an ophthalmologist or neurologist if you have a question.

Horner's Syndrome

Horner's syndrome is a lesion in the sympathetic pathway to the eye and may be caused by a lesion in the central, preganglionic, or postganglionic neuronal pathways.

The patient shows features of miosis and slight ptosis of the upper and lower eyelid on the affected side. If branches of the external carotid artery are affected, a loss of facial sweating (anhidrosis) occurs, and facial and conjunctival blood vessels may be dilated.

The diagnosis can be performed by using 0.4% cocaine on both eyes and observing the pupillary diameters 15 minutes later. The normal pupil dilates

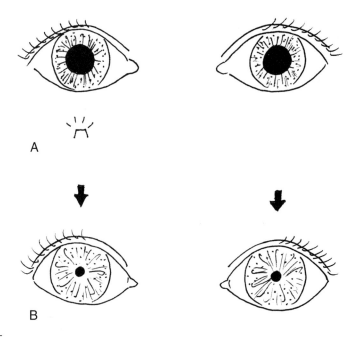

A

B

• **FIGURE 3–31**
Normal pupillary light reaction test. *A,* Direct response to light; result: constriction of stimulated pupil. *B,* Consensual response to light; result: constriction of contralateral pupil.

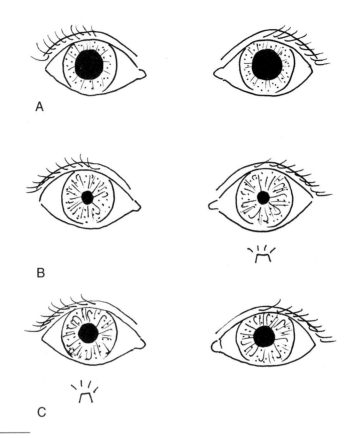

• FIGURE 3–32
Afferent pupillary defect (Marcus Gunn pupil). *A,* Diffuse illumination, both pupils equal in size. *B,* Light on normal left eye; result: normal constriction of both pupils. *C,* Light on eye with afferent defect; result: decreased reaction of both pupils.

and eyelids retract as reuptake of norepinephrine at the synapse is blocked by the cocaine. The diseased eye has no norepinephrine release to be blocked, and the pupil size does not alter. Failure to dilate to cocaine shows a postganglionic lesion. Preganglionic lesions include lesions such as Pancoast's tumor of the lung.

Examination and Management Summary

1. Perform the test for pupillary reaction at near and distance.

2. Is there an abnormal pupil light reflex?

3. Ascertain where the lesion might be in the pupillary light pathways.

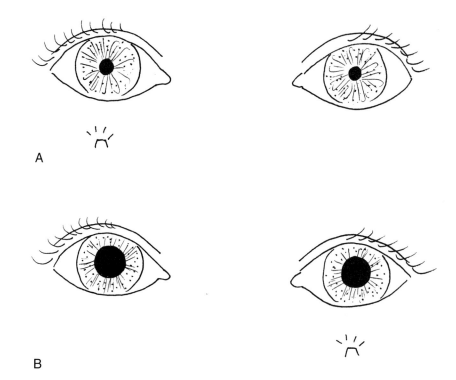

A

B

• **FIGURE 3–33**
Amaurotic pupillary response. *A,* Light on normal eye; result: constriction of contralateral pupil. *B,* Light on left eye, which is blind; result: constriction of contralateral pupil.

CATARACTS

The human lens changes size as the patient ages. The changes in size and coloration are part of the process of *cataract* formation, or cataractogenesis. The changes are classified as the opacification of the lens. These changes are seen in the cortex of the lens and in the nucleus of the lens (Figs. 3–34 and 3–35; see also Fig. 3–35 Color Plate 3).

Early lens changes can occur at age 50 or 60 years, but the patient may experience no change in visual acuity. In fact, the patient's visual acuity may be 20/20. However, as the lens changes progress, the patient may notice glare or "spokes" emanating from an oncoming headlight or street lamp. These optical aberrations now correspond to the patient's increasing lens changes inside the eye. When these optical aberrations cause diminished visual acuity and hamper the activities of daily living, such as reading or driving, cataract surgery is suggested.

Examination

The clinician, in using the direct ophthalmoscope, may not be able to see the optic nerve and retina as well as in previous examinations of the patient.

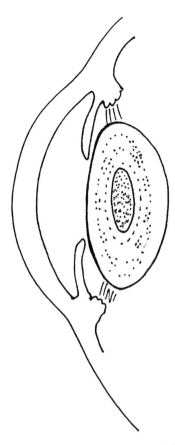

• **FIGURE 3–34**
Cataract (cross-section).

• **FIGURE 3–35**
Cataract.

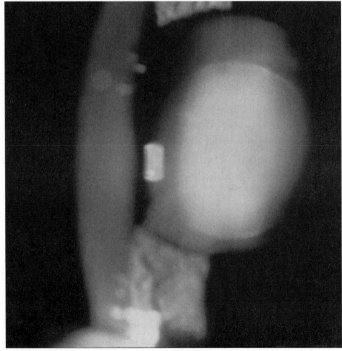

TABLE 3–13
CATARACT EVALUATION

1. Check the patient's vision with Snellen visual acuity assessment.
2. Can the patient perform the activities of daily living with this vision?
3. Can the patient see to drive, read, perform his or her occupation, and so on?
4. Refer the patient to an ophthalmologist for an evaluation.

In addition, by shining the direct ophthalmoscopic light in the patient's pupil, the clinician can discern a yellow discoloration of the lens (Table 3–13).

Treatment

Treatment is cataract surgery, which can be performed as an outpatient procedure, lasting up to an hour. An artificial intraocular plastic lens is inserted in the exact location of the previous lens (Fig. 3–36). Depending on the patient, glasses may or may not be needed after surgery. The success rate

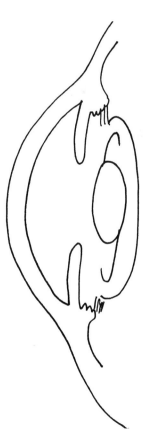

• **FIGURE 3–36**
Intraocular lens implant in capsular bag (cross-section).

of cataract surgery is 95% in patients without systemic disease, such as diabetes and hypertension, or ocular disease, such as glaucoma. In patients with a more complicated medical history, a discussion with the ophthalmologist is advised.

Examination and Management Summary

1. Check the patient's vision.

2. Look in with the direct ophthalmoscope to identify lens opacification or cataract if possible.

3. Refer the patient for cataract evaluation to an ophthalmologist who would perform surgery in the future.

4

Sudden Visual Loss

Loss of vision is a grave symptom in ophthalmology. It can occur in adults who are 40 to 80 years of age. Usually, the chief complaint involves (1) the loss of vision in one eye, (2) an abnormally constricted visual field, or (3) a large black or gray "veil," previously unseen, in the visual axis. The duration of the visual loss can be seconds or much longer.

The anatomy involved in visual loss is the eye and its vascular supply. The ophthalmic artery is derived from the first branch of the internal carotid artery. The first branches of the ophthalmic artery are the central retinal artery and the long posterior ciliary arteries. The retina is supplied by this vascular system and its anastomoses.

CENTRAL RETINAL VEIN OCCLUSION

Central retinal vein occlusion is a leading cause of sudden visual loss in elderly patients with hypertension, cardiovascular disease, or diabetes. Rarely, the underlying systemic cause is related to collagen vascular disease and hyperviscosity syndromes. The usual cause is a thrombosis of the central retinal vein in the area of the lamina cribrosa. Retinal vascular occlusion is second to diabetic retinopathy in causing severe visual loss (Table 4–1 and Fig. 4–1).

Patients with central retinal vein occlusion present with sudden visual loss. The fundal findings range from scattered hemorrhages and a few cotton wool spots to massive hemorrhages and massive retinal edema. The optic nerve may be edematous and surrounded by hemorrhages.

Treatment of systemic conditions is not effective in the management of ocular complications, although treatment of the underlying disorders may prevent the fellow eye from developing a central retinal vein occlusion.

No effective treatment exists. Laser photocoagulation is thought to help prevent ischemia of the retina and complications of neovascular glaucoma.

Patients' Description of Symptoms

Patients may describe having a sudden loss of vision that lasts for days, weeks, or months.

TABLE 4–1
RETINAL VASCULAR OCCLUSION MANAGEMENT

1. Test the patient's visual acuity with Snellen visual acuity.
2. Evaluate the patient for hypertension, diabetes, carotid artery disease, collagen vascular disease, and hyperviscosity syndromes.
3. Control of the systemic disease state in the patient may help prevent the disease in the fellow eye.
4. Refer the patient to an ophthalmologist.

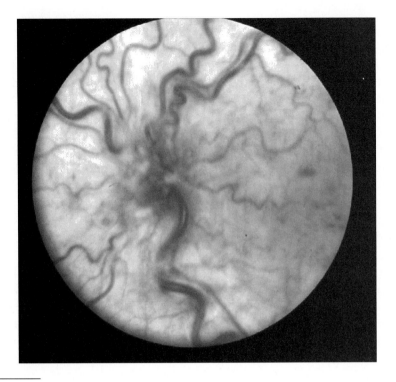

• **FIGURE 4–1**
Central retinal vein occlusion.

I can't see.

Everything went dark all of a sudden.

Last month, I started seeing blurry, then it went dark. I still can't see.

Patient's retinal findings include massive retinal hemorrhages that are easily seen with the direct ophthalmoscope. The optic nerve may be engorged and surrounded by hemorrhages.

Examination and Management Summary

1. The physician performs the Snellen visual acuity assessment: the patient's visual acuity is depressed.

2. The physician evaluates the patient for hypertension, diabetes, carotid artery disease, collagen vascular disease, and hyperviscosity syndromes; control of systemic disease helps prevent the disease in the fellow eye.

3. The patient is referred to an ophthalmologist, who may perform fluorescein angiography to determine the extent of the disease.

4. Laser therapy at the ophthalmologist's office.

Prognosis for Vision

The prognosis for vision in elderly patients with this disorder is poor. However, in the case of a young or middle-aged adult (30 to 40 years of age), the visual prognosis is better, but guarded.

BRANCH RETINAL VEIN OCCLUSION

Branch retinal vein occlusion affects males and females equally, typically between 60 to 70 years of age. The patient notices sudden blurred vision or partial occlusion of his or her visual field (see Table 4–1).

Vein occlusions occur at the site of arteriovenous crossings. Thus, arteriosclerotic changes occurring in that location have been postulated to lead to the branch retinal vein occlusion.

Hypertension, cardiovascular disease, and diabetes are associated closely with branch retinal vein occlusion (Fig. 4–2; see also Fig. 4–2 Color Plate 3).

Patients' Description of Symptoms

A sudden loss of vision occurs in part of the visual field, or a central dark spot is seen that has lasted for days, weeks, or months. Patients may present

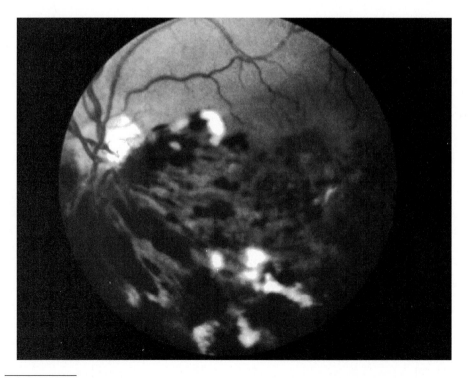

• **FIGURE 4–2**
Branch retinal vein occlusion.

with half of the visual field missing or may see the upper half or lower half of the world as black or gray.

> I see a black veil in front of my eyes. I've had this for a week.
>
> I see a small black spot when I read.
>
> I see only half my face in the mirror.
>
> When I look out the window, half of the window looks cloudy.
>
> I thought that my contact lenses/glasses were smudged. I can't see clearly. This has been going on for a month.

Examination and Management Summary

1. The patient presents with diminished visual acuity or partial loss of visual field.

2. The retinal findings show an area of retinal hemorrhages.

3. The ophthalmologist performs fluorescein angiography to help delineate the extent of the disease.

4. Treatment of the underlying systemic disease may not affect the course of the disease. However, control of the hypertension in affected patients may limit the ensuing central visual loss from retinal edema.

5. Laser treatment is thought to be helpful in the treatment of consequent retinal edema in branch retinal vein occlusion.

CENTRAL RETINAL ARTERY OCCLUSION

Although *central retinal artery occlusion* is rare, it deserves mention because the primary symptom is sudden loss of vision. Central retinal artery occlusion can be caused by emboli, intraluminal thrombosis, atherosclerotic plaques, vascular spasms, and vasculitis. Associated systemic diseases are arterial hypertension, diabetes mellitus, carotid atherosclerosis, and cardiac valvular disease (Fig. 4–3; see also Fig. 4–3 Color Plate 3; see Table 4–1).

Patients' Description of Symptoms

> At lunch, I just saw blackness, and I haven't been able to see anything since.
>
> I didn't have any pain, but I suddenly couldn't see out of my left eye.
>
> I haven't seen anything since Friday; that was 4 days ago.

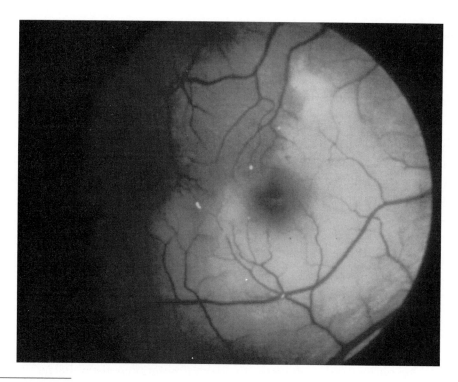

• **FIGURE 4–3**
Central retinal artery occlusion.

Examination and Management Summary

1. The patient can usually see only well enough to identify hand motion or count fingers.

2. The physician immediately refers the patient to an ophthalmologist or to an emergency department in which personnel are skilled in ophthalmologic care.

3. The ophthalmologist administers carbon dioxide treatment via face mask; this treatment is thought to dilate the retinal arterioles.

4. The ophthalmologist administers acetazolamide in order to lower the patient's intraocular pressure; this treatment is thought to decrease the resistance to blood flow in the retinal vessels.

5. The ophthalmologist administers ocular massage.

This treatment is successful in patients within the first few hours of the disease process.

Prognosis for Vision

If the patient has had the loss of vision for several days, the vision will remain poor. However, if the patient receives care by an ophthalmologist or emergency department personnel skilled in ophthalmologic care within a few hours of the onset of visual loss, the prognosis is better.

BRANCH RETINAL ARTERY OCCLUSION

Branch retinal artery occlusion has a pathophysiologic process that is similar to that of central retinal artery occlusion. Associated systemic diseases are hypertension, diabetes mellitus, carotid atherosclerosis, and cardiac valvular disease. Other, rarer causes are collagen vascular disorders, trauma, coagulopathies, and local ocular abnormalities (Fig. 4–4; see Table 4–1).

Patients' Description of Symptoms

Suddenly, I cannot see where my feet are.

There is a black spot in my vision when I read.

Examination and Management Summary

1. The vision may be 20/20 or less acute, but the patient has a visual field deficit that is diagnosed with confrontational visual fields.

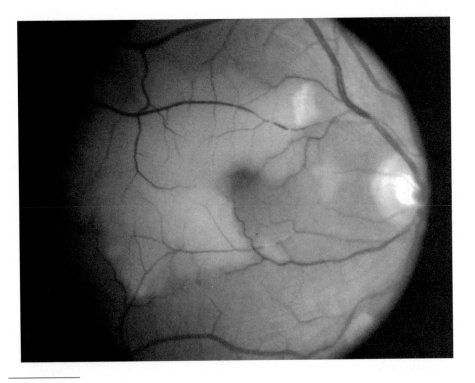

• **FIGURE 4–4**
Branch retinal artery occlusion.

2. The patient should be referred to an ophthalmologist, who would make the definitive diagnosis.

3. In branch retinal vein occlusion, no treatment exists, except for treatment of the underlying systemic disease. In some instances of branch retinal vein occlusion, laser therapy may be performed to improve the visual acuity if the disease process affects the central vision.

OTHER CAUSES OF VISUAL LOSS

The other cause of sudden visual loss is *retinal detachment and vitreous hemorrhage*, traumatic and diabetic (see Chapters 5 and 6). Although the incidence of retinal detachment is one in 10,000, this problem occurs with greater frequency in patients with myopia. Among myopes, the incidence of retinal detachment is thought to be 10 times higher. in young contact lens wearers or college-aged students who wear glasses for nearsightedness, loss of vision may be due to retinal detachment (Table 4–2).

The retina has certain areas of anatomic thinning at the junction of the retina and the iris. This area is called the pars plana region (Fig. 4–5; see

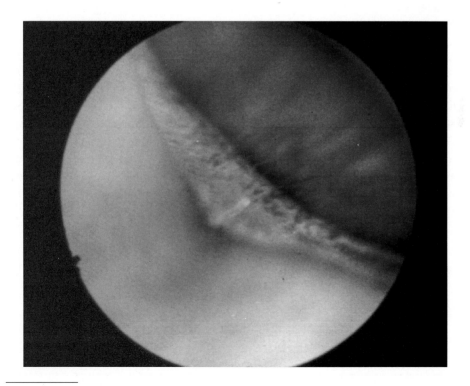

• FIGURE 4–5
Area of the pars plana in relation to the retina.

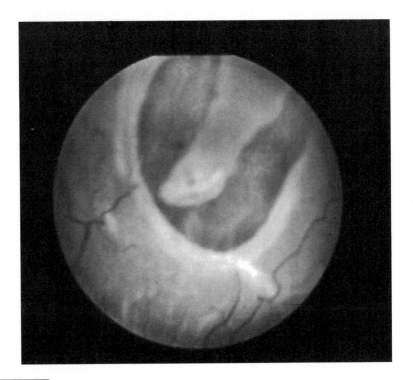

• **FIGURE 4–6**
Retinal hole.

also Fig. 4–5 Color Plate 4). In myopic eyes, these areas are stretched thinly over the circumference of the globe, and, in time, these thinned areas of the retina can develop a tear or a hole (Fig. 4–6). If that occurs, the retina detaches from its pigment layer, and a retinal detachment can occur (Figs. 4–7 and 4–8; see also Fig. 4–8 Color Plate 4). In young people, the vitreous, the gel inside the eye (Fig. 4–9), can support, or tamponade, a retinal hole for a long time; thus, a retinal detachment may not be discovered for a long time. In older adults, the vitreous is more liquid in consistency and cannot support the retina in its place; a retinal detachment occurs suddenly, and a subsequent loss of vision occurs.

TABLE 4–2

SUDDEN LOSS OF VISION

1. If decreased visual acuity or partial loss of visual field occurs, examine the patient with the direct ophthalmoscope.

2. If there is no view of the retina, refer the patient to an ophthalmologist.

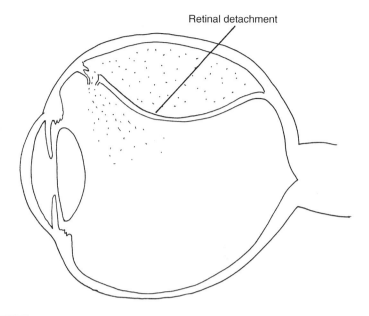

Retinal detachment

• **FIGURE 4–7**
Diagram of a retinal detachment, anteroposterior view.

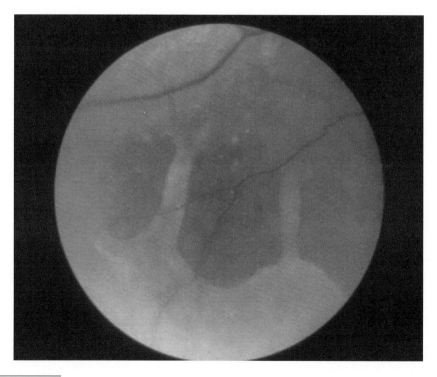

• **FIGURE 4–8**
Retinal detachment.

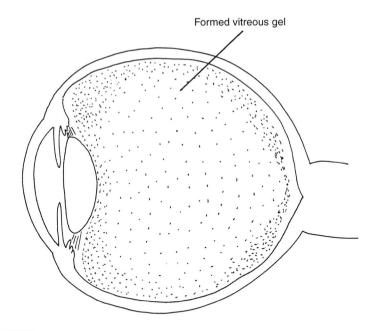

Formed vitreous gel

• **FIGURE 4–9**
Vitreous gel.

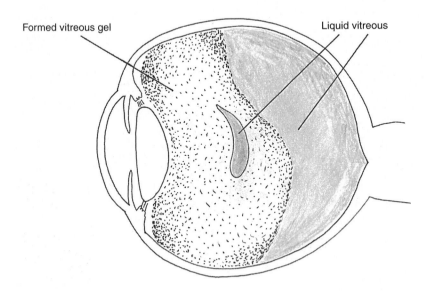

Formed vitreous gel

Liquid vitreous

• **FIGURE 4–10**
Posterior vitreous detachment.

TABLE 4–3
POSTERIOR VITREOUS DETACHMENT OR FLOATERS

1. The patient usually presents with a floater without pain or diminution of visual acuity.

2. The floater moves in the same direction as the eye movements.

3. Some floaters may lead to retinal detachment; therefore, a referral to an ophthalmologist is necessary.

Usually, retinal detachment occurs in adults, beginning from the third decade onward. It can also occur in the elderly after cataract surgery.

Patients usually note the onset of black floaters and flashes of light inside their eye; these phenomena are constant. An accompanying loss of vision then occurs in one quadrant of their vision.

Patients who experience chronic floaters have a posterior vitreous detachment (Fig. 4–10), where part of their vitreous gel becomes liquefied. The patient, in seeing the floater, is really seeing the optical interface between the vitreous gel and the vitreous liquid, as light enters the eye (Table 4–3). Unfortunately, a small percentage of these patients who experience floaters go on to have a retinal detachment. Therefore, all patients who experience floaters should see an ophthalmologist.

Patients' Description of Symptoms

Flashes, floaters, and loss or grayness of vision are common.

Last week, I saw some floaters. Then I saw flashes of light several times that day. The next day, I couldn't see out of my eye.

It seems that a window shade is pulled down partially in my eye.

When I look at my husband's face, the lower half of his face is out of focus and blurry.

Examination and Management Summary

1. The patient's visual acuity is decreased, or the visual field is partially lost.

2. Loss of the red reflex is observed by use of the direct ophthalmoscope. A white or gray reflex is present; the grayness is the detached retina.

3. The physician immediately refers the patient to an ophthalmologist or to an emergency department where the staff are skilled in ophthalmologic care.

4. Surgery is necessary for repair of the retinal detachment.

5. In certain cases, in which the retinal detachment is small and in the appropriate location, cryosurgery or laser surgery with the addition of intraocular gas injection can be performed in an outpatient setting.

5

Eye Emergencies Associated with Pain and Vision Loss

GLAUCOMA

Glaucoma is the leading cause of blindness in all age groups in the United States, but most commonly affects the elderly. Glaucoma is not a single disease process; rather, it is a large group of disorders characterized by widely diverse clinical and pathophysiologic processes. This fact is not well appreciated by the general public. One glaucoma patient has no pain and is treated with topical eyedrops, whereas another glaucoma patient suffers a painful angle closure glaucoma attack and is treated with emergency laser therapy. Thus, a spectrum of glaucoma patients with different presenting complaints exists.

Glaucoma is a condition in which intraocular pressure is too high for the normal functioning of the optic nerve. When damage to the optic nerve exists, the associated progressive loss of visual field occurs, leading to irreversible blindness. Thus, the parameters that ophthalmologists use to diagnose glaucoma are the intraocular pressure, the visual field, and the optic nerve.

Intraocular pressure deals with the production of aqueous humor by the ciliary body (behind the iris) and the outflow of the aqueous humor from the angle of the eye, which houses the trabecular meshwork and Schlemm's canal. The latter serves as a conduit to the venous drainage system near the surface of the eye. It is in the angle where the junction of the cornea meets the sclera that the classification of glaucoma lies (Figs. 5–1 and 5–2; see also Fig. 5–2 Color Plate 4).

Glaucoma is divided into *open angle glaucoma* and *closed angle glaucoma*. In open angle glaucoma, the angle appears anatomically normal to the naked eye, but the underlying trabecular meshwork, on a microscopic level, is abnormal, thus affecting its ability to drain the aqueous humor. As a result, the intraocular pressure is increased, causing damage to the optic nerve (Fig. 5–3; see also Fig. 5–3 Color Plate 4). In this type of glaucoma, the patient has no pain, just painless progressive loss of vision that is detectable by an ophthalmologist. Occasionally, as a harbinger for visual field loss, the patient experiences decreased vision in the dark or in twilight, suggesting loss of contrast sensitivity, which is one of the earliest signs of glaucoma. In advanced cases of glaucoma, severe visual field changes occur (Fig. 5–4). The treatment of open angle glaucoma involves the use of pharmaceutical agents that decrease the production of aqueous fluid, increase the drainage at the ciliary body, or a combination of the two. Laser has been used in patients whose intraocular pressure cannot be controlled on maximal medical therapy. Lastly, surgery is helpful in refractory cases or in advanced cases of glaucoma (Tables 5–1 and 5–2).

In *angle closure glaucoma* or *closed angle glaucoma*, the angle is narrowed anatomically such that the drainage of the aqueous fluid is impeded, resulting in an increase in intraocular pressure. In this instance, the patient has pain and/or nausea associated with this phenomenon. This type of glaucoma occurs in hyperopic individuals, in people who never wore glasses until

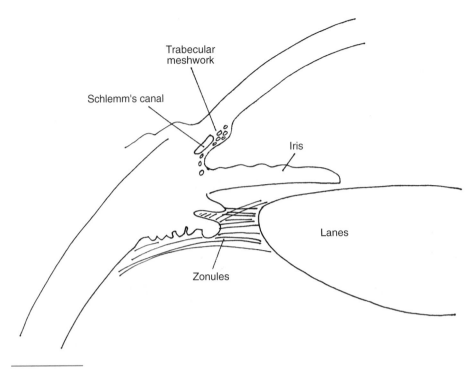

• **FIGURE 5–1**
The structures in the angle of the eye.

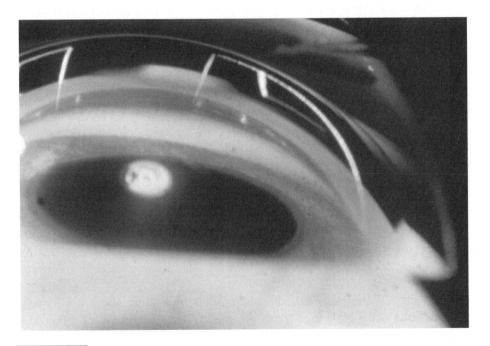

• **FIGURE 5–2**
Angle of the eye with fine neovascularization.

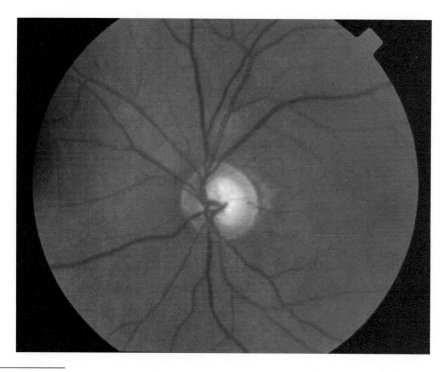

• **FIGURE 5–3**
Typical glaucomatous cupping. Note the hollowed-out appearance of the optic disc except for the thin border.

after the age of 40 years, or in people who have a family history of a "painful glaucoma episode." Treatment consists of the creation of an outflow pathway for the drainage of aqueous. This is commonly accomplished with laser surgery, although in rare cases, surgery may be necessary (Tables 5–3 and 5–4).

Open Angle Glaucoma

Patients' Description of Symptoms

I can't see to drive at night.

In a dark movie theater, I can't see to get to my seat as well as my wife.

My mother had to take eyedrops and became blind before she died.

My father had glaucoma, but he was very old. Do you think I could have it?

Examination and Management Summary

1. The physician obtains the pertinent family history and records the

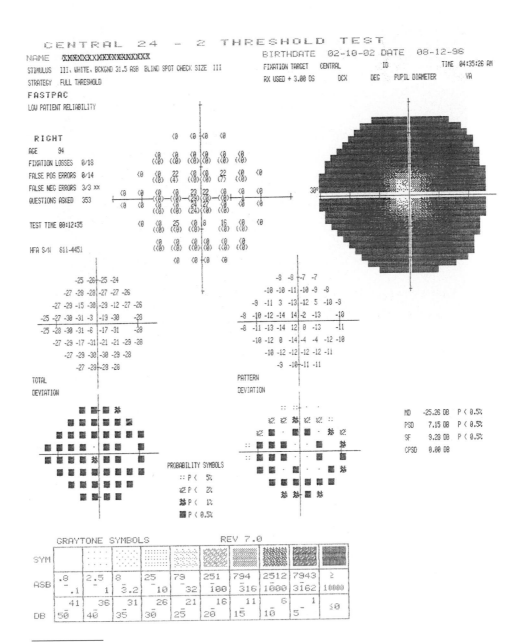

• **FIGURE 5–4**
Glaucomatous visual field loss, as documented with automated perimetry machine.

TABLE 5–1
OPEN ANGLE GLAUCOMA

1. Patient has painless, progressive visual loss.

2. Treatment is aimed at the lowering of intraocular pressure.

3. Glaucoma monitoring is performed by obtaining regular measurements of the patient's intraocular pressure and photographing the optic nerve and visual fields.

4. Nearly all blindness from glaucoma is preventable if detected early and properly treated.

TABLE 5–2
OPEN ANGLE GLAUCOMA MANAGEMENT

1. Obtain pertinent family history. If there is a positive family history, refer the patient to an ophthalmologist for evaluation.

2. Perform the Snellen visual acuity assessment.

3. Obtain a Schiøtz tonometer reading. Normal intraocular pressures are between 10 and 20 mm Hg.

4. Treatment is started by an ophthalmologist: topical eyedrops, e.g., timolol maleate.

TABLE 5–3
CLOSED ANGLE GLAUCOMA

1. Patient has pain, headache, nausea, and vomiting.

2. Moderate-to-severe visual loss can occur within hours.

3. The angle is narrowed anatomically, and there is poor drainage of the aqueous fluid resulting in increased intraocular pressure.

4. Immediate referral to the ophthalmologist is needed.

5. The ophthalmologist immediately performs laser treatment to the iris to create a new pathway for the drainage of aqueous.

TABLE 5–4
CLOSED ANGLE GLAUCOMA MANAGEMENT

1. Perform the Snellen visual acuity assessment (difficult to obtain in patients with severe pain).

2. Perform a penlight examination to ascertain the extreme redness of the eye and the lack of clarity of the cornea.

3. Refer the patient immediately to the ophthalmologist or nearest emergency department skilled in ophthalmologic care.

patient's symptoms. If the patient has a positive family history or suspicious symptoms, he or she is referred to an ophthalmologist for evaluation.

2. The physician performs the Snellen visual acuity assessment and watches the patient read. The physician determines whether the patient reads the whole line or drops off the end letters, suggesting a constriction of the visual field.

3. The physician performs a Schiøtz tonometer reading (Fig. 5–5). A drop of topical proparacaine is placed into the eye of the patient; then, the tonometer is placed on the cornea, as the patient is reclining. Disposable plastic covers are available to be used for this, or the Schiøtz

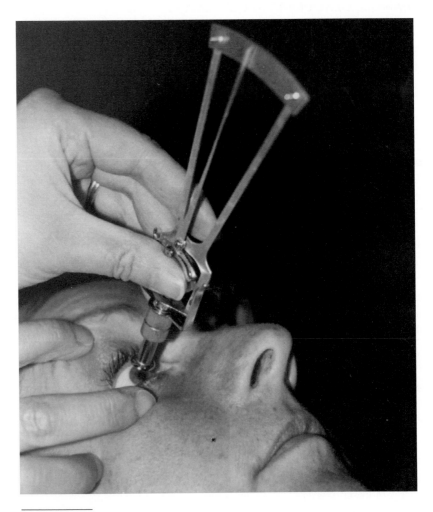

• **FIGURE 5–5**
Schiøtz tonometry reading.

tonometer can be sterilized for each patient. Normal intraocular pressures are 10 to 20 mm Hg.

4. The ophthalmologist starts treatment. In open angle glaucoma, the treatment is eyedrops, usually beta blockers, such as timolol maleate, which reduces aqueous production. Parasympathomimetics increase outflow facility. Parasympathomimetics in ophthalmology are direct-acting cholinergic agents, such as pilocarpine and carbachol. In addition, adrenergic agonists are available; these agents, which include epinephrine and its synthetic analogues, decrease aqueous production. Carbonic anhydrase inhibitors, such as acetazolamide, methazolamide, and dorzolamide, suppress secretion of the aqueous humor.

Closed Angle Glaucoma

Patients' Description of Symptoms

I have a mild headache, right over my eyebrows. I feel nauseated.

I can't see; I must have the flu because I have a headache and I want to vomit.

I have severe eye pain.

I have a headache, and I feel nauseated. Doctor, do you think it's my medications?

Examination and Management Summary

1. The physician obtains the pertinent family history and records the patient's symptoms.

2. The physician performs the Snellen visual acuity assessment. If the patient is in severe pain and will not open his or her eyes, the examination may be impossible.

3. If the patient can be examined, the physician can perform Schiøtz tonometry. The pressure is increased to greater than 20 mm Hg.

4. Penlight examination of the patient's eye shows some redness of the conjunctival area (see Chapter 1).

5. With the patient's eye closed, the physician uses his or her index fingers to palpate the eye and feel its ocular tension. If it feels rigid and unyielding, like a rock, the patient's intraocular pressure is very high, and the patient should be sent to an emergency department or to an ophthalmologist's office immediately.

6. The ophthalmologist obtains intraocular pressure readings with the use of the applanation tonometer of the slit-lamp biomicroscope (Fig. 5–6).

7. The ophthalmologist starts treatment. In closed angle glaucoma, if pain occurs, the treatment may be the use of eyedrops, acetazolamide tablets, liquid isosorbide, or intravenous mannitol. Laser surgery is performed to create a new outflow pathway for the aqueous. The timing of the laser surgery depends on the severity of the angle closure attack.

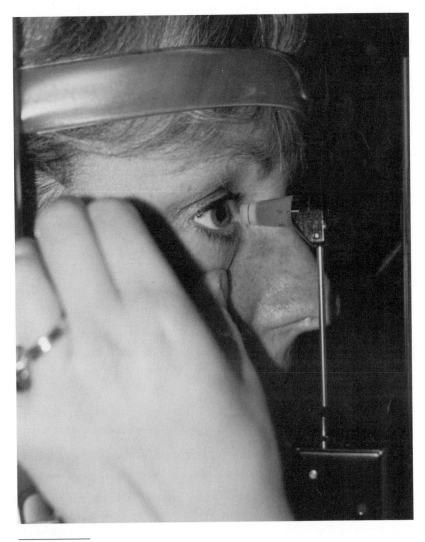

• **FIGURE 5–6**
Applanation tonometry at the slit lamp at the ophthalmologist's office.

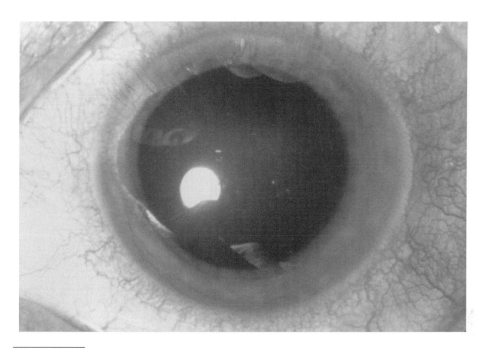

• **FIGURE 5–7**
Conjunctival injection from contact lens overwear.

PAIN AND CONTACT LENS USE

Pain can occur in patients who wear contact lenses. Pain can be caused by overwear or excessive wearing time of the contact lens. These patients present with a red eye with mild-to-moderate conjunctival injection (Fig. 5–7; see also Fig. 5–7 Color Plate 4). In other instances, the pain can be due to a piece of dust caught under the contact lens. This situation can cause severe pain. Other times, rubbing the eye with the contact lens in place can cause pain (Table 5–5).

Hard contact lenses and soft contact lenses can cause the same problems.

TABLE 5–5

MANAGEMENT OF CONTACT LENS–INDUCED PAIN

1. If the soft contact lens is still in the eye, try to flush out the lens by irrigating copiously with sterile saline.

2. If the hard contact lens is still in the eye, copious irrigation may or may not work. If it fails, refer the patient to an ophthalmologist immediately.

3. Once the contact lens is out of the eye, instill ophthalmic erythromycin antibiotic ointment and then pressure patch the eye (see Fig. 3–2).

4. Refer the patient to an ophthalmologist for follow-up.

It is important for the physician to ask if the problem is related to contact lens usage.

Patients' Description of Symptoms

> I have severe pain, and I can't open my eye. I think my contact lens is not fitting right.

> I slept in my contact lens, and I can't open my eyes.

> I feel something in my contact lens.

> Usually, I don't feel my contact lens, but today, I feel uncomfortable.

Examination and Management Summary

1. The physician performs the Snellen visual acuity assessment. Testing visual acuity in the patient with pain may be difficult.

2. The physician looks at the eye with a penlight. Sometimes, the contact lens problem can be seen.

3. The physician instructs the patient to remove his or her contact lens.

4. The physician uses a fluorescein strip to determine whether a corneal abrasion is present. A specially designed penlight with a blue filter is available at low cost at optical houses.

5. If a corneal abrasion is present, the physician can pressure patch the eye with two eye pads (see Fig. 3–2). First, a small amount of topical ophthalmic antibiotic ointment, such as bacitracin or erythromycin ophthalmic ointment, is added. Then, the physician folds over one eye pad and places the next eye pad on top. These eye pads are placed over the closed eyelids of the patient. The tape is placed in a diagonal fashion, from the forehead to the zygoma. Several strips of tape are placed, such that the entire eye pad is covered with tape.

6. The physician refers the patient for follow-up with an ophthalmologist the next day.

TRAUMA

Trauma to the eye can result in eye pain and/or visual loss. Eye trauma is the leading cause of severe visual loss in children and adolescents. Many of the incidents can be prevented by goggles and other protective eyewear.

Trauma to the eye is extremely common during sports activities. School children are poked in the eye while playing basketball, causing a minor injury. This type of injury causes iritis, an inflammation of the iris that leads to the release of prostaglandins. These cell mediators are thought to be part of the ocular inflammation. Slight pain and photophobia can occur. Treatment is with topical steroids or nonsteroidal anti-inflammatory agents. Blunt trauma can cause retinal edema, "commotio retinae" (Fig. 5–8; see also Fig. 5–8 Color Plate 4). This edema resolves spontaneously, and good vision returns.

Other patients are hit in the eye with a baseball or tennis ball, which can cause fracture of the orbital bones surrounding the eye or rupture of the eyeball itself. Sometimes, orbital fractures involve damage to the nasal passages and sinuses, and the patient has difficulty breathing. Ice hockey injuries to people who were not wearing facemasks have caused devastating trauma to the eye (Fig. 5–9; see also Fig. 5–9 Color Plate 5). These injuries cause damage to the internal ocular tissues, such as the retina and the vitreous. The blunt injury can cause the vitreous gel inside the eye to reverberate and rub against the retina, causing severe damage. The retina can be torn, and a retinal detachment can ensue (Fig. 5–10; see also Fig. 5–10 Color Plate 5). Alternatively, the vitreous reverberation can lead to a rupture of blood vessels inside the eye, leading to a vitreous hemorrhage. The eyeball may look normal, but in actuality, serious damage may have occurred inside the globe

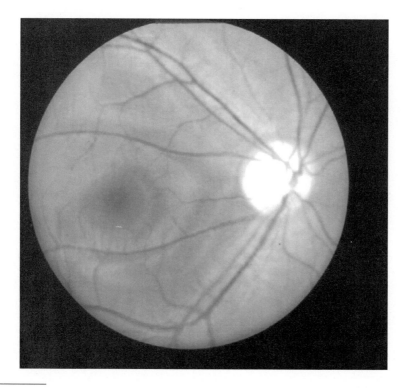

• **FIGURE 5–8**
Retinal edema from blunt trauma to the eye.

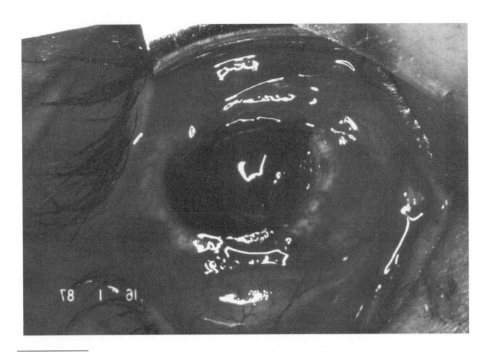

• **FIGURE 5–9**
Ruptured globe.

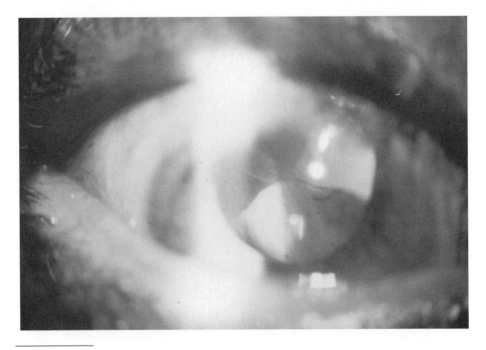

• **FIGURE 5–10**
Extruded lens in a ruptured globe resulting from severe trauma to the eye. (Courtesy of Lory Snady-McCoy, MD, Providence, RI.)

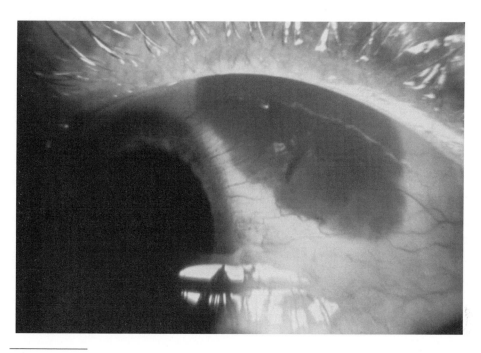

• **FIGURE 5–11**
Scleral laceration from penetrating injury.

(Fig. 5–11; see also Fig. 5–11 Color Plate 5). The vision is severely impaired in these cases.

In severe trauma to the eye, the patient has a swollen eye. It is obvious that he or she should be seen in an emergency department, experienced in ophthalmologic care, immediately.

Other trauma from a penetrating foreign body, such as a pellet gun or a metal nail in a toy toolbox, may result in an injury to the globe (Fig. 5–12; see also Fig. 5–12 Color Plate 5). In these cases of ruptured globe, the eye may look normal except for a small red hemorrhage at the conjunctiva, indicating an entrance wound of a penetrating foreign body (Fig. 5–11; see also Fig. 5–11 Color Plate 5). Because a foreign body penetration is highly suspected, tetanus antitoxin should be considered. In these cases of penetrating injury, the ophthalmologist should be consulted immediately. The physician team members may begin administering antibiotics systemically.

In other instances of eye trauma, the eyelids are opened and the eye looks anatomically normal (Fig. 5–11; see also Fig. 5–11 Color Plate 5); however, the vision is poor, and the patient experiences general eye pain or pain when looking at lights (photophobia). The patient may complain of flashes and floaters and an inability to see out of the traumatized eye. In this instance, the physician should consider the presence of retinal detachment or blood inside the eye, involving the vitreous (Fig. 5–13; see also Fig. 5–13 Color Plate 5). Alternatively, the patient may have a vitreous hemorrhage and

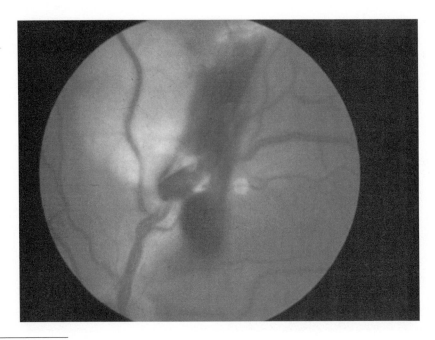

• **FIGURE 5–12**
Penetrating injury to the eye with intraocular metallic foreign body lodged in the retina.

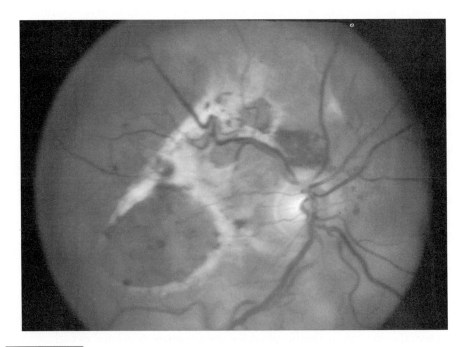

• **FIGURE 5–13**
Scarring of the retina caused by blunt trauma to the eye.

TABLE 5–6
TRAUMA MANAGEMENT

1. Perform the Snellen visual acuity assessment.
2. Perform a penlight examination.
3. Do not force the eye open.
4. Administer tetanus immunization.
5. Refer the patient to an ophthalmologist for follow-up.

blood in the anterior chamber (hyphema) and have glaucoma and increased intraocular pressure (Tables 5–6 and 5–7 and Fig. 5–14; see also Fig. 5–14 Color Plate 5).

Patients' Description of Symptoms

I can't see, and the light bothers me.

After I got hit with the baseball, I've seen little black floaters.

My eye looks red and it hurts. I have a headache, and I want to vomit.

After the ball hit me, my eye turned black and blue and I breathed funny.

Examination and Management Summary

1. The physician performs the Snellen visual acuity assessment. If the eye is swollen shut, the physician should not force the eyelids open. Instead, the patient should be referred to an ophthalmologist.

2. If the patient can be tested and the vision is severely depressed with

TABLE 5–7
TRAUMA PREVENTION

1. Use goggles or protective eyewear for sports.
2. Do not allow young children or toddlers to play with sharp objects.
3. Avoid projectile toy guns, which can be dangerous for all ages.

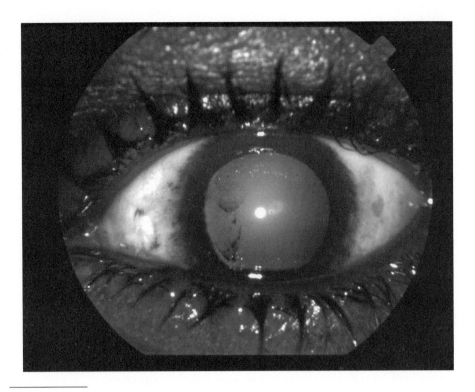

• **FIGURE 5–14**
Blood in the anterior chamber and glaucoma from traumatic injury to the globe.

respect to his or her fellow eye, the patient should be referred to an ophthalmologist.

3. The physician should examine the patient with a penlight and inspect the eye.

4. If the physician has lingering questions, the patient should be referred to an ophthalmologist.

5. In cases of pain, nausea, vomiting, and headache, the patient should be immediately referred to an ophthalmologist or to an emergency department skilled in ophthalmologic care.

6

Systemic Disease

DIABETES

Diabetic Retinopathy

Diabetic retinopathy is the leading cause of blindness in Americans 20 to 64 years of age. Although only 4% of the diabetic population has the severe type of proliferative diabetic retinopathy, many more Americans are affected with minor variations of the disease process in their eyes.

Diabetic eye disease can affect all parts of the eye: the cornea, the iris, the lens, and the retina. In the cornea, diabetes manifests itself as poor healing after trauma or inability to tolerate contact lens wear. In the iris, diabetic patients show iris atrophy (Fig. 6–1; see also Fig. 6–1 Color Plate 6), and slight changes are seen in the ophthalmologist's office. Diabetic patients are prone to development of open angle glaucoma and neovascular glaucoma (Fig. 6–2; see also Fig. 6–2 Color Plate 6), in which large blood vessels grow on the iris. Diabetic patients can show cataractous lens changes earlier than the fourth or fifth decade of life, different from age-matched control patients. In the retina, the changes can be minor to severe, but all begin with the pathologic abnormality associated with hyperglycemia: loss of endothelial cell function of the vasculature. Thus, the retinal vessels leak blood or lipid (Fig. 6–3; see also Fig. 6–3 Color Plate 6) or form saccular outpouchings or dilations and tortuosities (Fig. 6–4; see also Fig. 6–4 Color Plate 6). Alternatively,

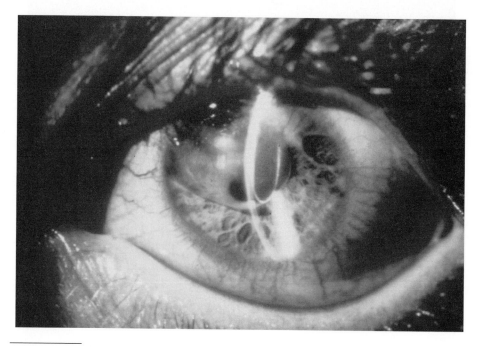

• **FIGURE 6–1**
Iris atrophy.

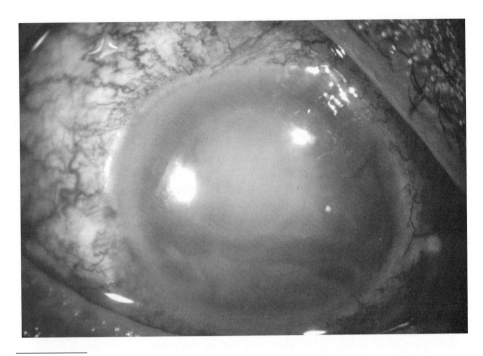

• **FIGURE 6–2**
Neovascular glaucoma.

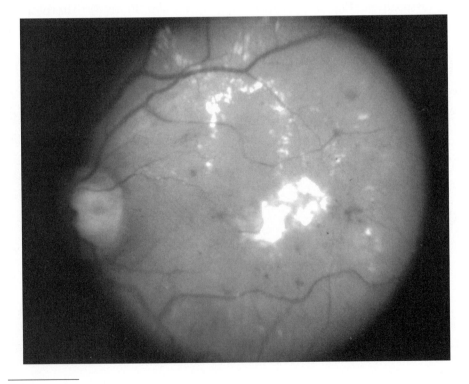

• **FIGURE 6–3**
Hard exudates from diabetic retinopathy.

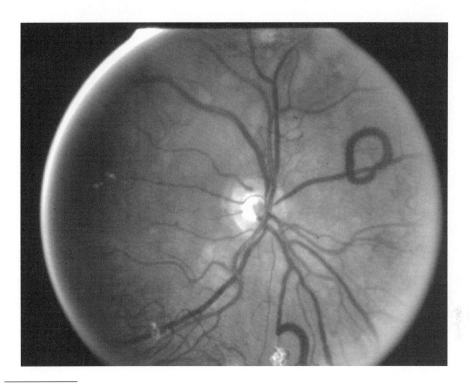

• **FIGURE 6–4**
Venous loop.

the retinal vessels form areas of neovascularization, which are thin-walled abnormal vessels that leak blood and are a sign of generalized retinal ischemia and inadequate blood flow and oxygenation to the vital parts of the eye (Fig. 6–5; see also Fig. 6–5 Color Plate 6).

Commonly, the diabetic patient may complain of poor vision or a small dark shadow in the middle of the page while reading (*macular edema*) (Fig. 6–6). Other times, in a patient with insulin-dependent (type 1) diabetes, the patient complains of sudden visual loss (vitreous hemorrhage) (Fig. 6–7; see also Fig. 6–7 Color Plate 6). Yet on other occasions, the patient is asymptomatic, but the physician finds *cotton wool spots* (Fig. 6–8; see also Fig. 6–8 Color Plate 7), *dot blot hemorrhages* (Fig. 6–9; see also Fig. 6–9 Color Plate 7), or *hard exudates* (Fig. 6–10; see also Fig. 6–10 Color Plate 7).

The classification of diabetic retinopathy has become more detailed in the past decade as a result of the Early Treatment Diabetic Retinopathy Study, funded by the National Institutes of Health.[1] In the beginning of the disease process, no diabetic retinopathy exists; this stage is classified as *no diabetic retinopathy* (Table 6–1 and Fig. 6–11; see also Fig. 6–11 Color Plate 7).

Later in the development of the disease is a stage in which just a few microaneurysms (<30) (Fig. 6–12; see also Fig. 6–12 Color Plate 7) to

Text continued on page 104

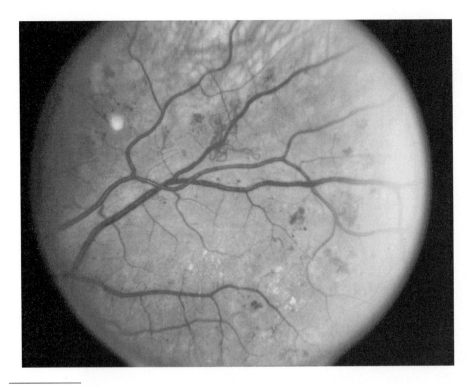

• **FIGURE 6–5**
Retinal neovascularization.

AMSLER RECORDING CHART

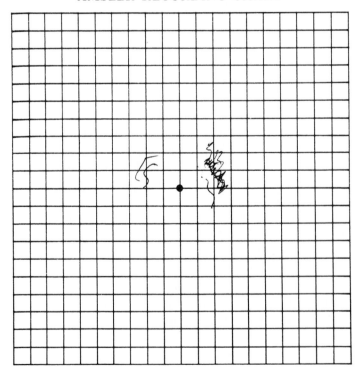

• **FIGURE 6–6**
Amsler grid showing area of decreased vision for the patient.

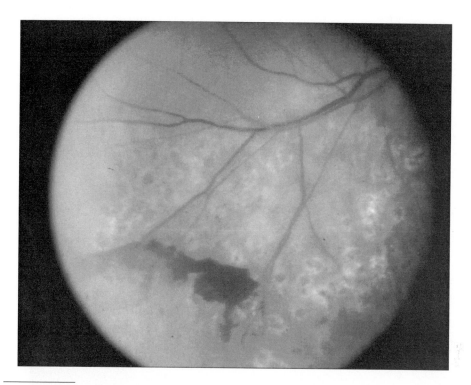

• **FIGURE 6–7**
Vitreous hemorrhage.

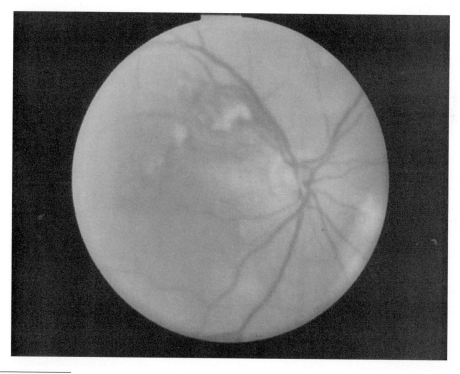

• **FIGURE 6–8**
Cotton wool spot.

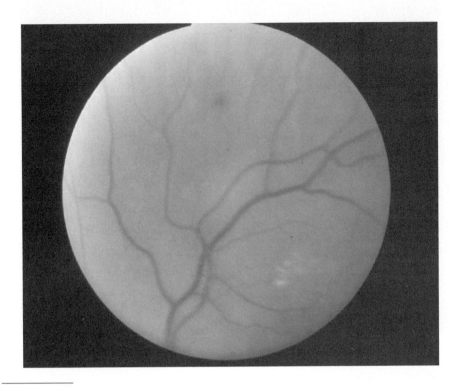

• **FIGURE 6–9**
Dot hemorrhages in background diabetic retinopathy.

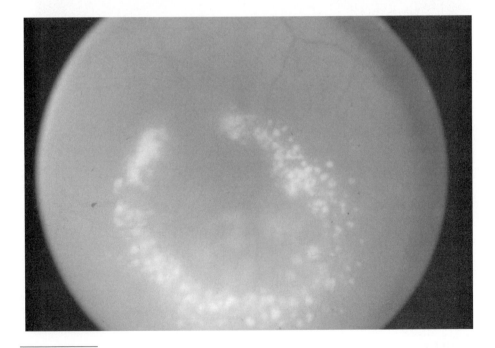

• **FIGURE 6–10**
Hard exudates.

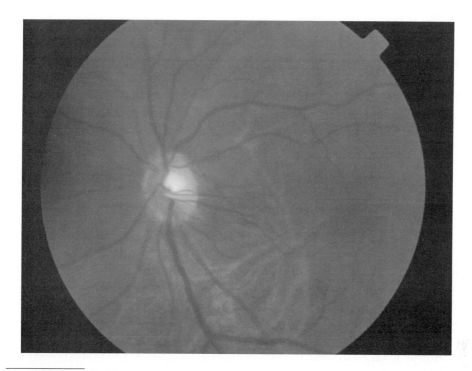

• **FIGURE 6–11**
No diabetic retinopathy.

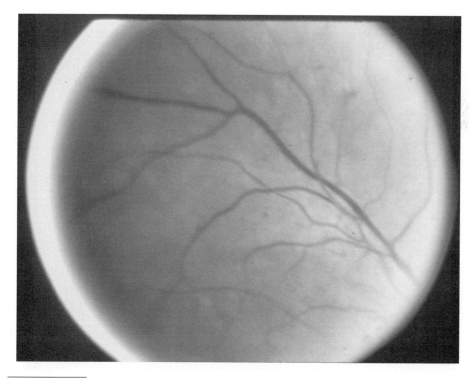

• **FIGURE 6–12**
Background diabetic retinopathy with fewer than 30 microaneurysms.

TABLE 6–1

NO DIABETIC RETINOPATHY

1. Perform the Snellen visual acuity assessment.

2. Look at the patient's iris for iris neovascularization.

3. Examine the patient's retina with the direct hand-held ophthalmoscope. Observe the optic disk margins and the macula.

4. If you have any questions, consult with an ophthalmologist. If any blood or hard exudates are seen, refer the patient to an ophthalmologist.

numerous microaneurysms are present, with changes in venous caliber; this is called *nonproliferative diabetic retinopathy* (Fig. 6–13; see also Fig. 6–13 Color Plate 7). This stage was formerly known as background or preproliferative diabetic retinopathy (Table 6–2). In this stage, referral to an ophthalmologist is necessary because the rate of change for the disease is unpredictable.

At any stage of diabetic retinopathy, macular edema can occur (Table 6–3 and Fig. 6–14; see also Fig. 6–14 Color Plate 8). Macular edema occurs when microvascular leaking occurs in the macula, the part of the retina that provides the precise vision of 20/20 or the appreciation for fine details and

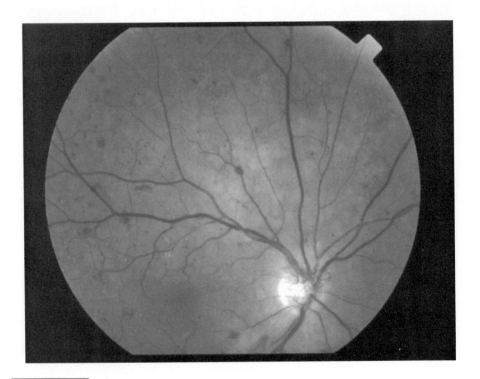

• **FIGURE 6–13**
Nonproliferative diabetic retinopathy.

TABLE 6–2

NONPROLIFERATIVE DIABETIC RETINOPATHY

1. Perform the Snellen visual acuity assessment.

2. If multiple areas of small dot blot hemorrhages, hard exudate, cotton wool spots, or venous tortuosity are seen, refer the patient to an ophthalmologist for an evaluation.

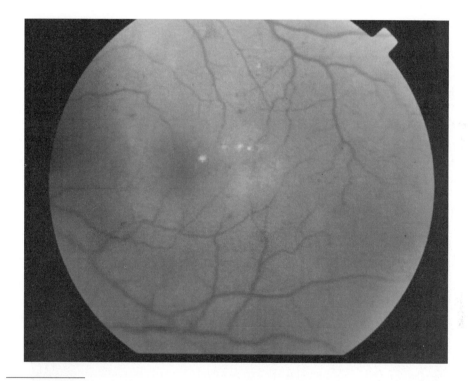

• **FIGURE 6–14**
Mild diabetic macular edema.

TABLE 6–3

MACULAR EDEMA

1. Perform the Snellen visual acuity assessment.

2. Hard exudates and pinpoint microaneurysmal bleeding suggest the presence of macular edema.

3. Refer the patient to an ophthalmologist for possible laser therapy.

color. The end capillaries become blunted or form small outpouchings called *microaneurysms*, thus making the cone cells in the retina function abnormally. In addition, the leakage of proteins and blood products into the retinal cells displaces their normal anatomic placement and causes distortion in the central vision (Fig. 6–15; see also Fig. 6–15 Color Plate 8). This phenomenon is common in patients with non–insulin-dependent (type 2) diabetes mellitus, who may have not seen an ophthalmologist regularly and are seeking a change in their spectacle correction. Unfortunately, health care providers must tell such patients that their underlying disease process is causing this change in vision. Referral to an ophthalmologist is necessary. Early laser intervention has been found to be useful in maintaining useful vision for these patients.

The most severe stage of diabetic retinopathy is known as *proliferative diabetic retinopathy* (Table 6–4). It is at this stage that the patient is at high risk for severe visual loss. The patient shows signs of new vessel growth on the retina, experiences sudden visual loss from a vitreous hemorrhage (Fig. 6–16; see also Fig. 6–16 Color Plate 8), and, lastly, may have a traction retinal detachment. Traction retinal detachments occur when the vitreous overlying the retina contracts because of bleeding or new vessel growth (Fig. 6–17; see also Fig. 6–17 Color Plate 8). Subsequently, an anteroposterior force pulls the

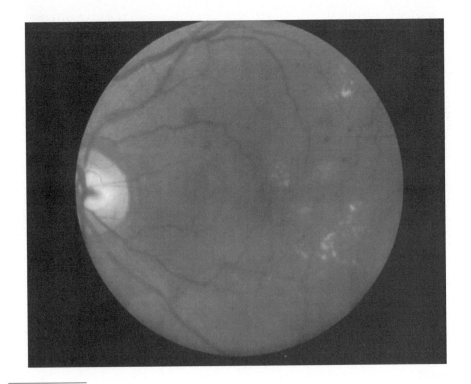

• FIGURE 6–15
Diabetic macular edema, with changes associated with nonproliferative diabetic retinopathy.

TABLE 6–4
PROLIFERATIVE DIABETIC RETINOPATHY

1. Perform the Snellen visual acuity assessment.
2. Large areas of hemorrhage are observed all over the retina.
3. The view of the retina may be hazy secondary to a vitreous hemorrhage.
4. Refer the patient to an ophthalmologist for evaluation and treatment.

retina away from its underlying layers. Thus, a retinal detachment ensues—a dreaded complication of diabetic retinopathy (Fig. 6–18; see also Fig. 6–18 Color Plate 8). Although the most severe stage of diabetic retinopathy exists in only 4% of the diabetic population, proliferative diabetic retinopathy is the most common indication for diabetic eye surgery involving the retina.

At the ophthalmologist's office, additional testing, such as fluorescein angiography, may be performed (Fig. 6–19). This test involves the injection of a fluorescein dye intravenously into the arm of the patient while the patient is seated at a camera. The camera is equipped with specially colored filters, which show the autofluorescence of the dye as it reaches the patient's retinal

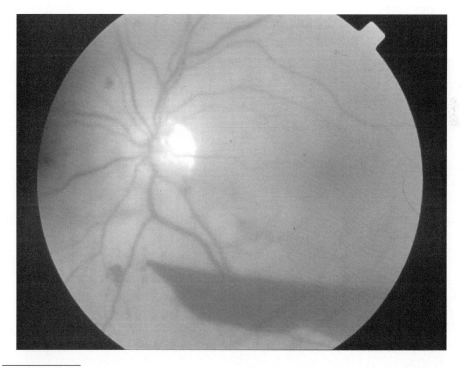

• **FIGURE 6–16**
Diabetic vitreous hemorrhage.

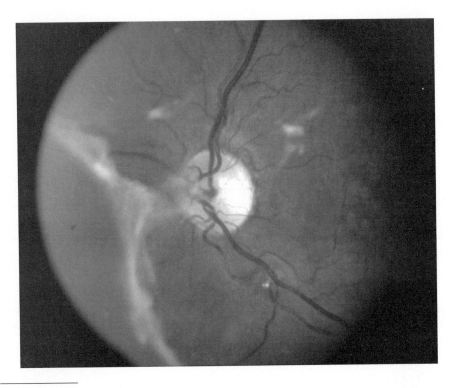

• **FIGURE 6–17**
Mild diabetic traction retinal detachment.

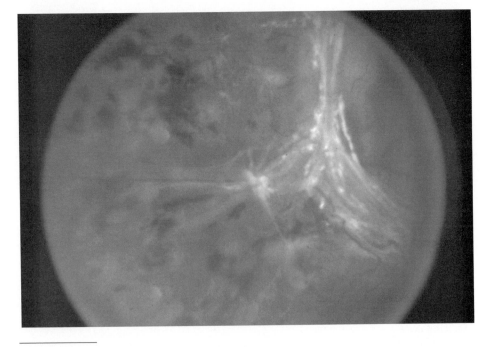

• **FIGURE 6–18**
Severe diabetic traction retinal detachment.

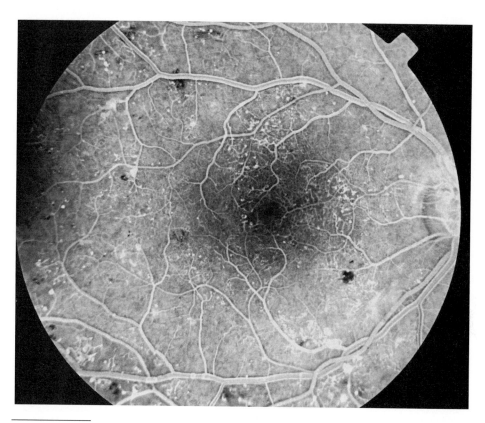

• FIGURE 6–19
Fluorescein angiogram of diabetic macular edema.

vessels. The transit time for the dye is approximately 15 to 20 seconds. This test allows the ophthalmologist to detect macular edema and areas of diabetic retinopathy not easily seen by the ophthalmologist.

Another test that may be performed is ultrasonography of the eye (Fig. 6–20). This test is important for the detection of a retinal detachment when a vitreous hemorrhage is present. It is part of the evaluation of a patient with a vitreous hemorrhage because an occult retinal detachment would require surgery.

Laser surgery is common for diabetic patients. Laser is the abbreviation for light amplification by stimulated emission of radiation. The stimulated emission of light from excited atoms or molecules is amplified and is thus a powerful, monochromatic, directional beam of light. In ophthalmology, the light is used to deliver small pulses of energy at millisecond intervals to control areas of bleeding or new vessel growth in diabetes (Fig. 6–21; see also Fig. 6–21 Color Plate 8).

Microsurgery on the retina and the vitreous is necessary for the treatment of proliferative diabetic retinopathy when the patient has a long-standing vitreous hemorrhage or retinal detachment. This type of surgery typically

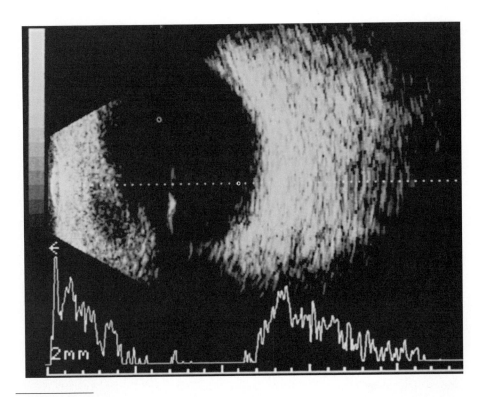

• **FIGURE 6–20**
Ultrasonogram showing vitreous hemorrhage.

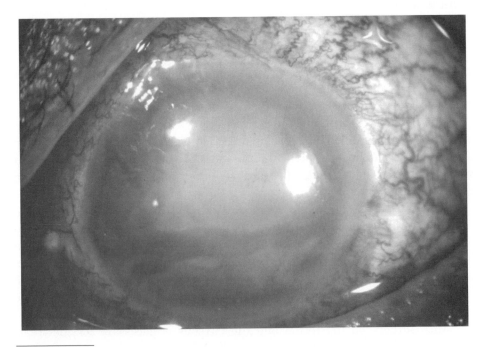

• **FIGURE 6–21**
New vessels on the iris and hyphema in the anterior chamber.

takes place in a hospital or ambulatory surgical setting. The instruments are all very small and are mechanized and activated by foot pedal action. These instruments are used under a surgical microscope, and the patient undergoes general or local anesthesia for the procedure.

Patients' Descriptions of Symptoms

No Diabetic Retinopathy

I've had diabetes for 10 years, and I see pretty well. I haven't had an eye check-up for 10 years. Should I see an ophthalmologist, Doctor?

My father went blind from diabetes. Should I be tested even though my blood sugar control is good?

Nonproliferative Diabetic Retinopathy

There's a black spot in the middle of my page whenever I read.

The car lights don't seem as bright in my left eye as in my right eye.

The world looks smudgy in spots.

Macular Edema

The lines on the newspaper are wavy.

As I read, some of the letters are not on the same line. They seem smaller than the letter next to it.

I look at the walls in my house, and some of the walls look wavy.

I can't pass the driver's license test.

I bought four different pairs of glasses, and none of them work. I still can't see up close.

I can't see to sign my checks.

Proliferative Diabetic Retinopathy

I was doing fine until yesterday, when I saw huge black lines dripping inside my eye. I kept thinking it would go away but it hasn't.

I woke up, and I couldn't see out of my left eye.

I was lifting my luggage and suddenly, one eye saw funny.

In the past, I have had many lasers in my eye, and suddenly, I can't see out of my eye today.

My vision was bad in my right eye, but suddenly, I can't see out of my left eye, my good eye.

My doctor told me I had a problem with my left eye but that it would be okay after laser surgery, but now, I can hardly walk around in my apartment.

Examination and Management Summary

1. The physician performs the Snellen visual acuity assessment for distance and near vision.

2. The physician watches the patient read the eye chart and determines whether the patient misses certain letters in each line, for example, does he or she miss the left letters on all of the lines or the central letters?

3. The physician looks at the patient's iris and looks for any traces of red, which would be evidence of new vessels on the iris (Fig. 6–21).

4. The physician looks inside the patient's retina with the direct handheld ophthalmoscope and observes the optic disk margins and the macula.

5. If the physician has any questions, he or she calls an ophthalmologist.

6. If any blood or hard exudates are seen, the patient is referred to an ophthalmologist; hard exudates and pinpoint microaneurysmal bleeding suggest the presence of macular edema. The ophthalmologist would consider fluorescein angiography and laser treatment to the focal areas of leakage.

7. If new blood vessels are on the iris, the retina, or the optic disk, laser treatment would be the next step in most cases.

8. If there is no view of the retina and the eye is filled with blood in the vitreous cavity, laser treatment and/or surgery may be the next option.

Other Forms of Diabetic Eye Disease

CORNEAL DISEASE

The diabetic patient has *abnormal corneal epithelium* as a result of the loss of integrity of the tight junctions between the epithelial cells. In addition, diabetic patients have a loss of corneal sensitivity. Diabetic patients with long-standing diabetes commonly have dry eye or minor problems of the anterior surface of the eye. All of these characteristics of the diabetic cornea lead to its inability to heal properly. Thus, a simple corneal abrasion can develop into a corneal ulcer, or the same small corneal abrasion can take days to weeks to heal properly (Table 6–5).

Patients' Description of Symptoms
I am a diabetic, and I have had a red eye for several days.

My red eye went away; now, I have a white spot on my eye and I can't see, but I have no pain.

TABLE 6–5
DIABETIC CORNEAL PROBLEMS

1. Patient has tearing or dry eye, despite therapy with artificial tears.
2. Patient is intolerant of contact lens use.
3. Patient has persistent pain in the front of the eye.
4. Patient has persistent or recurrent corneal abrasions.
5. Refer the patient to an ophthalmologist for further evaluation.

> I have had a red eye for a week. I think something got in my eye, but it has been hurting me for 4 days.

Examination and Management Summary

1. The physician performs the Snellen visual acuity assessment for distance and near vision.

2. The physician looks at the cornea with a penlight and determines whether the light reflex is abnormal.

3. If the physician has any questions, he or she refers the patient to an ophthalmologist for evaluation.

4. The ophthalmologist examines the patient with a slit-lamp biomicroscope.

5. If a corneal abrasion is present, the ophthalmologist may patch the eye or use a bandage contact lens and apply topical antibiotic eyedrops.

GLAUCOMA

Open angle *glaucoma* is associated with diabetes mellitus (Table 6–6) for reasons that are unclear. Thus, diabetic patients need yearly examinations for glaucoma. Open angle glaucoma leads to painless, progressive visual loss.

TABLE 6–6
OPEN ANGLE GLAUCOMA IN DIABETIC PATIENTS

1. Glaucoma is associated with diabetes.
2. Refer patients with diabetes and a family history of glaucoma to an ophthalmologist for further evaluation.
3. Otherwise, yearly examinations for glaucoma should be performed by an ophthalmologist.

TABLE 6–7
NEOVASCULAR GLAUCOMA

1. Perform the Snellen visual acuity assessment.

2. Look at the patient's iris for any traces of red, which would be evidence of iris neovascularization.

3. Take an intraocular pressure reading with the Schiøtz tonometer.

4. If you have any questions, call an ophthalmologist.

Neovascular glaucoma or hemorrhagic glaucoma occurs in diabetic patients entering the proliferative stage of their disease process (Table 6–7 and Fig. 6–22). New vessel growth occurs anteriorly toward the anterior segment of the eye and eventually leads to new vessel growth posteriorly toward the retina. This type of new vessel growth anatomically clogs up the eye's drainage mechanism, the trabecular meshwork. The intraocular pressure increases, causing minor eye pain and minor headache pain. Sometimes, the patient's intraocular pressure increase may take weeks or months to occur after the first observation of red vessels on the iris of the eye.

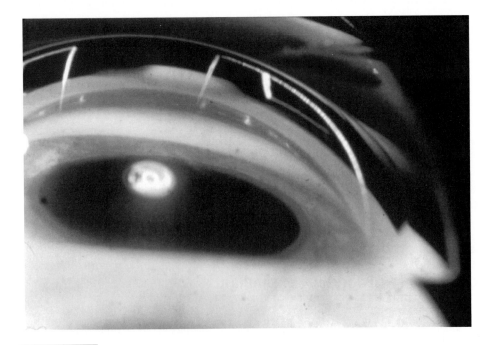

• **FIGURE 6–22**
New vessels in the angle.

Patients' Description of Symptoms

My blue eyes look funny: one of them has a pinkish tinge to it.

I have had a headache over my right eye for several weeks.

Examination and Management Summary

1. The physician performs the Snellen visual acuity assessment for distance and near vision.

2. The physician looks at the patient's iris for any traces of red, which would be evidence of new vessels on the iris.

3. The physician takes an intraocular pressure reading with the Schiøtz tonometer.

4. If the physician has any questions, the patient can be referred to an ophthalmologist.

5. If eye pressure is increased, the physician calls an ophthalmologist for advice and referral.

6. If there are discernible pink vessels on the patient's iris, the patient is referred to an ophthalmologist for further evaluation and treatment.

7. The usual treatment for neovascular glaucoma is lowering of the intraocular pressure with topical medications (see Chapter 5) and using laser surgery to eradicate the new vessels in the retina. Sometimes, the management of the elevated intraocular pressure is difficult, and glaucoma surgery may be necessary.

HYPERTENSION

Systemic hypertension is associated with vascular lesions in the eyes. Elevated blood pressure causes focal and generalized constriction of the retinal arterioles mediated by autoregulation. Prolonged duration of particularly high blood pressure can be associated with breakdown of the inner blood-retina barrier, with extravasation of plasma and red blood cells, retinal hemorrhages, cotton wool spots, intraretinal lipid, closure of retinal capillaries, and occlusion of the blood supply to the retina (Fig. 6–23).

Diffuse arteriolar narrowing is a hallmark of hypertensive retinopathy, a cause in the decrease in the arteriole-to-venule ratio from the normal ratio of 2:3. The focal narrowing is thought to be due to local edema in the wall of the arteriole or to areas of fibrosis (Table 6–8 and Fig. 6–24). A progressive increase occurs in the elastic component of the intima of the arteriole, and an

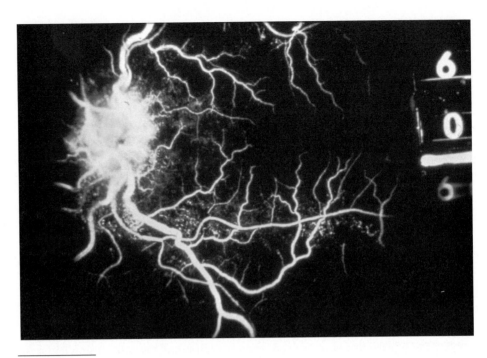

• **FIGURE 6–23**
Fluorescein angiogram of malignant hypertension.

increase occurs in the collagen component of the muscularis layer. The changes in the walls of the arterioles change the character of the light reflex from the vessels.

Atherosclerotic changes occur in the intima of the larger vessels. Lipid deposition occurs in the intima and is associated with calcification and fibrosis. Such changes have been seen in the peripapillary retinal arteries and the choroidal arteries (Table 6–9).

Hypertensive optic nerve changes can occur with accelerated hypertension. The cause of the these changes is not clear.

TABLE 6–8

THE SCHEIE CLASSIFICATION OF HYPERTENSION

Stage 0: No changes.
Stage I: Diffuse, uniform arteriolar narrowing.
Stage II: Arteriolar narrowing is both more prominent and focal.
Stage III: Both focal and diffuse arteriolar narrowing and retinal hemorrhages are present.
Stage IV: Stages I–III with retinal edema, hard exudates, and papilledema.

Scheie H: Evaluation of ophthalmoscopic changes of hypertension and arteriolar sclerosis. Arch Ophthalmol 49:117–125, 1953.

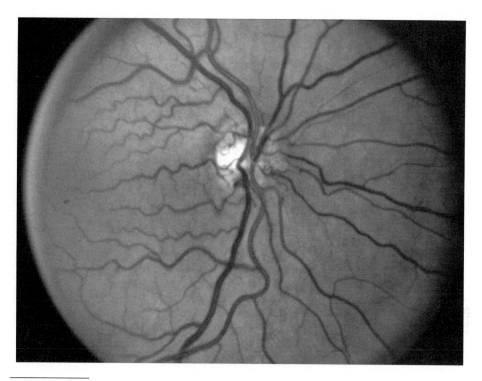

• **FIGURE 6–24**
Arteriosclerotic changes in the vessels in hypertension.

Patients' Description of Symptoms

I have a severe headache, and I can't see well enough to read.

I have a central spot in my vision.

I can't see the way I used to see.

I suddenly can't see out of my right eye.

TABLE 6–9
THE SCHEIE CLASSIFICATION OF ARTERIOSCLEROSIS

Stage 0: Normal.
Stage I: Broadening of the arteriolar light reflex with minimal or no arteriolovenous changes.
Stage II: Light reflex and arteriolovenous crossing changes are more obvious.
Stage III: "Copper wire" arterioles.
Stage IV: "Silver wire" arterioles and arteriolovenous crossing changes are most severe.

Scheie H: Evaluation of ophthalmoscopic changes of hypertension and arteriolar sclerosis. Arch Ophthalmol 49:117–125, 1953.

Examination and Management Summary (Table 6–10)

1. The physician performs the Snellen visual acuity assessment.

2. The physician examines the patient's optic nerve.

3. If there are changes in the blood vessels such as those described in the Scheie classification, the physician may consider referral to the ophthalmologist.

4. The physician regulates the patient's hypertension.

5. The physician refers the patient to an ophthalmologist to evaluate the patient's vision and retinal findings. Sudden loss of vision in the patient necessitates immediate referral to an ophthalmologist.

LEUKEMIA AND OTHER HEMATOLOGIC MALIGNANCIES

Most patients with chronic *leukemias* have intraocular involvement at the time of death. Minor problems related to the eyes can occur frequently. Most commonly, after chemotherapeutic regimens, patients experience a sensation of dry eyes or "grittiness" in their eyes. During chemotherapy, many patients experience a generalized fatigue of their bodies and an inability to focus at distance or read, despite appropriate spectacles. This is related to a divergence insufficiency and a generalized inability to concentrate and focus on small print.

On routine ophthalmic examinations, patients with leukemia can manifest small areas of bleeding in the periphery of the retina. Because the lesion does not affect the macula, the patients may never have a complaint. Usually, these areas of localized bleeding resolve, and monitoring of their blood count and platelets is sufficient (Figs. 6–25 and 6–26; see also Figs. 6–25 and 6–26 Color Plate 7). In addition, there are small lesions called white-centered hemorrhages in which a collection of white blood cells is surrounded by a

---

TABLE 6–10

HYPERTENSIVE RETINOPATHY MANAGEMENT

1. Perform the Snellen visual acuity assessment.

2. Evaluate the patient's optic nerve, looking for disk edema, hemorrhages, or retinal edema.

3. Continue monitoring the patient's hypertension.

4. Refer the patient to an ophthalmologist if there is sudden loss of vision or if severe hypertensive retinopathy is seen.

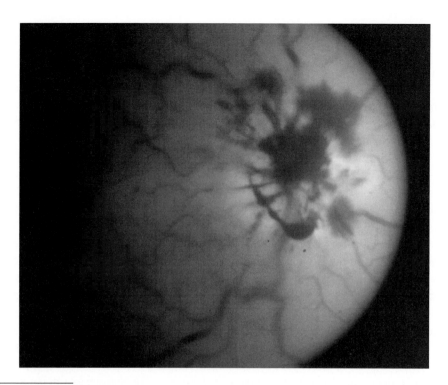

• **FIGURE 6–25**
Optic nerve hemorrhage in acute lymphocytic leukemia.

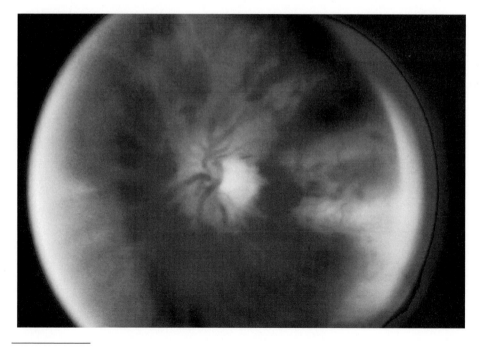

• **FIGURE 6–26**
Retinal hemorrhages in acute lymphocytic leukemia.

small hemorrhage. Lastly, patients with leukemia may also manifest neovascularization, which consists of areas of fine, abnormal new vessels, like those seen in patients with diabetes. Cotton wool spots can occur as well.

More severe eye changes occur when the patient complains of loss of vision or blurriness of vision in one eye. In this situation, serous retinal detachment may be overlying choroidal infiltrates or choroidal masses. Vitreous hemorrhages can also rarely occur.

In moribund patients, vitreous infiltrates have been found (Fig. 6–27; see also Fig. 6–27 Color Plate 7). The veins and arteries may develop a yellowish tinge because of the anemia and massive number of cotton wool spots. Whole blood hyperviscosity may lead to venous occlusive disease, microaneurysm formation, retinal hemorrhages, and retinal neovascularization.

The patient with leukemia can manifest various neuro-ophthalmic problems. An isolated nerve palsy of the third, fourth, fifth, sixth, or seventh nerve may occur. In these cases, any central nervous system problems concomitant to the patient's disease should be documented with computed tomography or magnetic resonance imaging. When the isolated nerve palsies occur, an acute onset of diplopia may occur. Temporary treatment is a patch over one of the eyes so that the patient may function monocularly in his or her immediate environment. The ophthalmologist provides temporary prism glasses in order to alleviate the patient's diplopia. The temporary prisms can

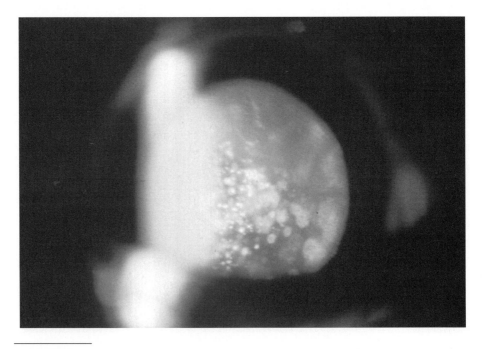

• FIGURE 6–27
Vitreous infiltrates in acute lymphocytic leukemia.

be cut out and pasted to the patient's eyeglasses and changed as the patient's diplopia changes during the course of his illness.

Patients' Description of Symptoms

My eyes feel dry and uncomfortable.

I can't read at all. By the way, I am taking chemotherapy for my leukemia.

I can't focus when I look at something far away or something nearby.

I can't see out of one eye.

I see double.

Examination and Management Summary

1. The physician performs the Snellen visual acuity assessment.

2. The physician looks to see that the pupils are equal and reactive.

3. The physician checks the extraocular movements and facial movements for third, fourth, fifth, sixth, and seventh nerve palsies.

4. The physician looks with the direct ophthalmoscope for any cotton wool spots, bleeding, or other abnormalities.

5. If the physician has questions, he or she calls an ophthalmologist for advice. If the patient has loss of vision or diminished visual acuity, prompt referral to an ophthalmologist is needed. If the patient has diplopia from an isolated eye muscle palsy, referral to an ophthalmologist is advised.

6. If the patient has a dry eye sensation, over-the-counter tear substitutes are a good remedy. Prescription tear medications are available as well.

7. If the patient has a loss of focusing ability, the physician refers him or her to an ophthalmologist.

8. If the patient has a loss of isolated cranial nerve function, the physician refers him or her to an ophthalmologist or a neurologist. The ophthalmologist may need to prescribe prism glasses for this period.

9. If the patient has a loss of vision, the patient is referred immediately to an ophthalmologist (Table 6–11).

LYMPHOMA

The incidence of intraocular involvement in patients with *lymphoma* is approximately 6%.

TABLE 6–11
EYE DISEASE AND SYSTEMIC ONCOLOGIC DISEASE MANAGEMENT

1. Perform the Snellen visual acuity assessment.

2. If the patient has dry eye sensation from chemotherapeutic agents, prescribe artificial tears.

3. If the patient has visual loss or neurologic deficit, refer him or her to an ophthalmologist or a neurologist, respectively.

NON-HODGKIN'S LYMPHOMA

Retinal hemorrhages and cotton wool spots related to anemia or thrombocytopenia are common in *non-Hodgkin's lymphoma*. Rarely, perivenous infiltrates are found and are treated with radiation (Table 6–11 and Fig. 6–28; see also Fig. 6–28 Color Plate 9).

HODGKIN'S LYMPHOMA

Cotton wool spots; Roth's spots, or white-centered hemorrhages; retinal hemorrhages; chorioretinitis; perivascular retinitis; or exudative retinal de-

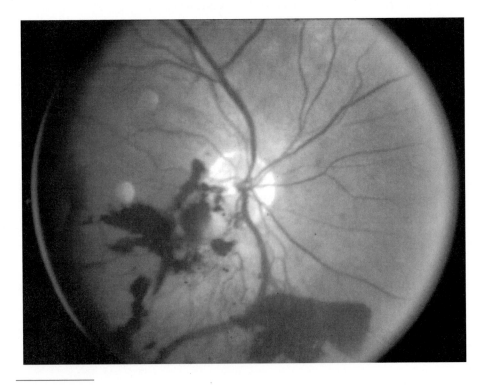

• **FIGURE 6–28**
Retinal hemorrhages in Hodgkin's lymphoma.

tachments are commonly seen in *Hodgkin's lymphoma*. Patients also have cells in the anterior chamber and in the vitreous.

MULTIPLE MYELOMA AND WALDENSTRÖM'S MACROGLOBULINEMIA

The intraocular manifestations of *macroglobulinemia* are anemia and thrombocytopenia. Flame-shaped or white-centered hemorrhages and cotton wool spots are seen. Microaneurysm formation may be seen in the retinal periphery. Hyperviscosity changes can present with venous obstructive disease, microaneurysms, and peripheral retinal neovascularization.

Patients' Description of Symptoms

I cannot see very well; I just had treatment for lymphoma.

I woke up and I couldn't see my face in the mirror.

I can't read clearly.

The world looks hazy to me.

Examination and Management Summary

1. The physician performs the Snellen visual acuity assessment.

2. Occasionally, the patient can see only well enough to identify hand motion or count fingers.

3. The physician looks inside the retina to identify the optic nerve head and the macula. The physician looks for cotton wool spots or hemorrhages, as well as for vascular abnormalities.

4. The physician refers the patient to an ophthalmologist for further evaluation. There may be lesions in the retina.

5. If the ophthalmoscopic findings are positive, then the primary care physician and oncologist confer jointly about systemic treatment.

METASTATIC DISEASE

Metastatic disease to the choroid occurs because of its vascularity. The choroid is the most common site for intraocular metastases. Metastatic choroidal tumors are yellowish or whitish-yellow. Usually, associated serous retinal detachment is present that may be out of proportion to the metastatic mass lesion.

For females, most metastatic disease to the eye is caused by breast carcinoma. Less commonly, bronchogenic carcinoma and gastrointestinal malignancy can metastasize to the choroid in females. In males, the most common primary tumors are lung, kidney, gastrointestinal tract, testicular, and prostate, in decreasing order of frequency.

Evaluation of the metastatic lesion in the ophthalmologist's office includes the examination of the fellow eye because metastatic disease can be bilateral. Evaluation of the lens is useful because radiation therapy may be cataractogenic. For diabetic patients with microvascular abnormalities, documentation of the pre-existing eye lesions is necessary because radiation exacerbates the microangiopathy.

Fluorescein angiography may be performed to assess the size of the metastatic lesion. Ultrasonography is used to determine the size of the mass lesion. In patients with media opacities or retinal detachments, the ultrasonography is useful to ascertain any mass lesions.

Although most patients present with history of known primary tumor, the evaluation of the metastatic disease depends on the previous extent of testing. Additional testing with computed tomography or magnetic resonance imaging is necessary to determine the extent of central nervous system involvement. In addition, it is important to assess the other metastases in the skeletal system and other organ systems (Table 6–11).

Patients' Description of Symptoms

I see floaters.

My vision is blurred.

I see double and triple images.

I have pain in my eye.

My eye is red, and I have floaters.

I am missing part of my face when I look in the mirror.

Examination and Management Summary

1. The physician performs the Snellen visual acuity assessment. Poor visual acuity may suggest metastatic activity in the retina.

2. The physician tests the pupils to ascertain the presence of central nervous system involvement.

3. The physician examines the optic nerve, areas of the retina, and the macula.

4. If the physician suspects ophthalmic involvement, the patient is referred to an ophthalmologist for further evaluation.

5. The ophthalmologist reports the extent of the eye findings to the primary care practitioner and the oncologist, and a treatment plan is determined.

ACQUIRED IMMUNODEFICIENCY SYNDROME

Ocular involvement occurs in up to 70% of patients with *acquired immunodeficiency syndrome* (AIDS), with the most common lesions being noninfectious retinopathy, such as cotton wool spots. Common ocular manifestations of AIDS are cotton wool spots, cytomegalovirus retinitis, retinal hemorrhages, Kaposi's sarcoma of the conjunctiva, keratitis sicca, cranial nerve paralysis, and papilledema, in decreasing order of frequency.

Cotton wool spots are a result of the microinfarction of the nerve fiber layer of the retina (Fig. 6–29; see also Fig. 6–29 Color Plate 9). Isolated retinal hemorrhages are also seen in patients with AIDS.

Cytomegalovirus retinitis can occur in half of all AIDS patients. The patients present with hemorrhage and cotton wool spots (Fig. 6–30; see also Fig. 6–30 Color Plate 9) associated with necrosis along the vasculature

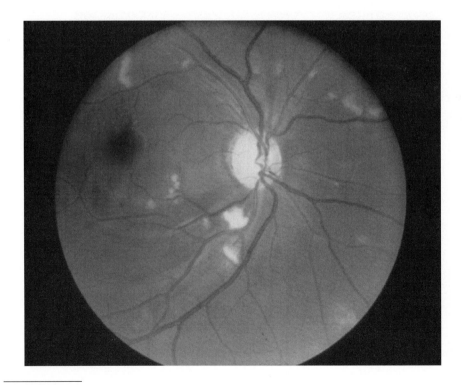

• **FIGURE 6–29**
Cotton wool spots in the acquired immunodeficiency syndrome.

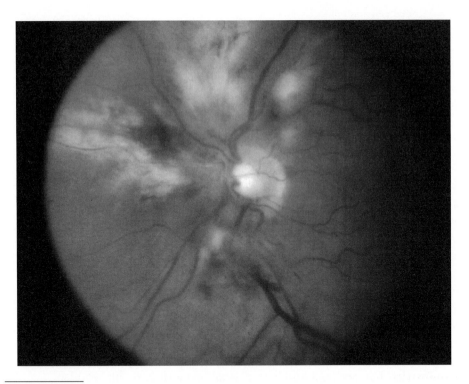

• **FIGURE 6–30**
Cytomegalovirus retinitis with cotton wool spots.

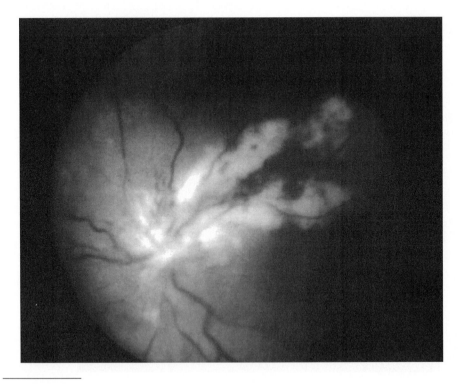

• **FIGURE 6–31**
Cytomegalovirus retinitis with necrosis along the vasculature.

(Fig. 6–31; see also Fig. 6–31 Color Plate 10). An intense whitening of the retina occurs; this is the necrotizing retinitis of the cytomegalovirus infection (Fig. 6–32; see also Fig. 6–32 Color Plate 10).

Acute retinal necrosis can occur, with associated retinal detachment and loss of vision. The etiologic agent is thought to be within the herpesvirus family.

Kaposi's sarcoma of the conjunctiva presents as a vascularized purplish lesion in the conjunctival area, seen when the eyelid is drawn down to expose the conjunctiva (Fig. 6–33; see also Fig. 6–33 Color Plate 10). It can range in size from only a few millimeters to large-mass 10-mm lesion.

Dry eye or keratitis sicca can occur in patients with AIDS, although the exact etiologic process is unclear; these conditions are symptomatically treated with artificial tear replacements.

Cranial nerve palsies can occur, signaling central nervous system involvement.

Optic disk edema can occur as a type of optic neuritis. Papilledema can occur as a result of elevated intracranial pressure, again demonstrating central nervous system involvement (Table 6–12 and Fig. 6–34; see also Fig. 6–34 Color Plate 10).

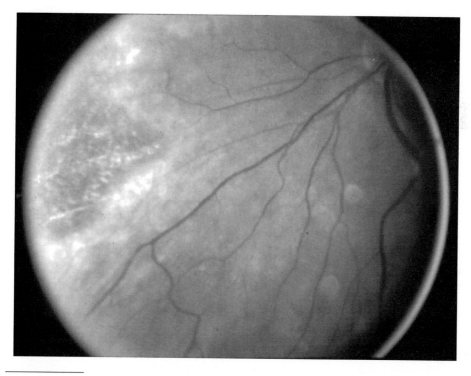

• **FIGURE 6–32**
Regressed cytomegalovirus retinitis.

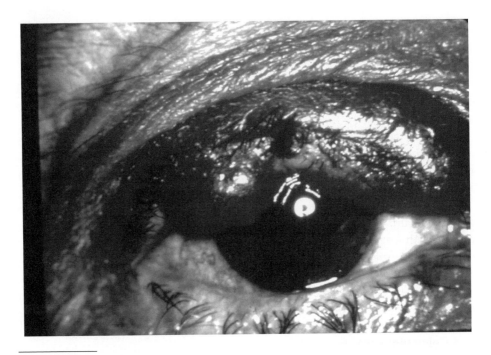

• **FIGURE 6–33**
Kaposi's sarcoma.

Patients' Description of Symptoms

I cannot see.

I have lost half of the upper field of vision.

There is a central black spot in my reading vision.

I see floaters.

Examination and Management Summary

1. The physician obtains the history and laboratory tests results of the
   T-cell counts.

TABLE 6–12
ACQUIRED IMMUNODEFICIENCY SYNDROME MANAGEMENT

1. Perform the Snellen visual acuity assessment.

2. Look for Kaposi's sarcoma.

3. If the patient has acute or chronic visual loss, refer him or her to an ophthalmologist.

4. The primary care physician performs routine follow-up with the ophthalmologist in
   concordance with changes in the T-cell count of the patient.

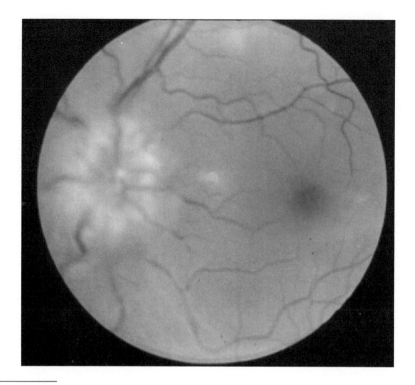

• **FIGURE 6–34**
Optic nerve edema with associated cotton wool spots in acquired immunodeficiency syndrome.

2. The physician performs the Snellen visual acuity assessment.

3. The physician performs a pupillary examination.

4. The physician views the cornea and the conjunctiva, looking for Kaposi's sarcoma.

5. The physician views the optic nerve and the macula.

6. The physician refers the patient to an ophthalmologist when there is acute or chronic visual loss.

7. The primary care physician performs routine follow-up in concordance with changes in the patient's T-cell count.

8. The ophthalmologist reports the extent of the eye findings to the primary care practitioner and infectious disease specialist to determine the appropriate systemic treatment plan.

9. If the patient has visual loss, or if areas of the retina are involved, thereby threatening sight, the ophthalmologist may offer treatment options such as the injection of antiviral agents into the eye via

surgery or the implantation of various slow-release gels impregnated with antiviral agents. Antiviral agents used for local ophthalmic injection are foscarnet and ganciclovir.

Reference

1. Early Treatment Diabetic Retinopathy Study Group. Early Treatment Diabetic Retinopathy Study. Report Number 1. Photocoagulation for diabetic macular edema. Arch Ophthalmol 103:1796–1806, 1985.

7

Optic Nerve Disorders

Patients with abnormalities of the optic nerve may present to the primary care practitioner's office in a variety of ways. Most commonly, the patient presents with the nonspecific complaints of a headache and mild changes in vision or transient obscuring of vision. Severe visual loss can occur slowly, over time.

PAPILLEDEMA

Papilledema is optic disk swelling caused by increased intracranial pressure (Fig. 7–1; see also Fig. 7–1 Color Plate 10). It is almost always bilateral, without visual acuity disturbances. According to one theory for the pathogenesis of papilledema, increased cerebrospinal fluid around the optic nerve head is transmitted in the optic nerve sheaths with associated stagnation of venous return from the retina and the optic nerve head. The obstruction to venous return gives the picture of dilated retinal veins, exudates, hemorrhages, and cotton wool spots, which are infarcts of the nerve fiber layer. Another theory suggests that the increased intracranial pressure causes a compression of the optic nerve fibers in the subarachnoid space of the intraorbital portion of the optic nerve. The blockage of the intra-axonal fluid mechanics causes a leakage

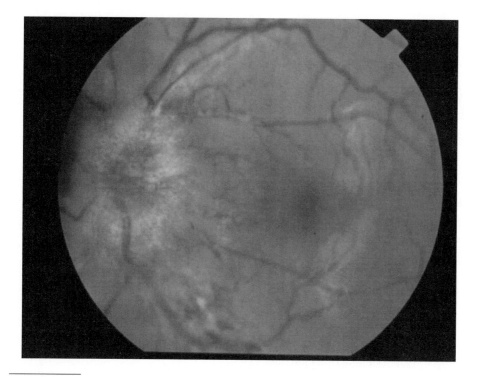

• **FIGURE 7–1**
Papilledema.

of water, protein, and axoplasmic contents into the extracellular space of the prelaminar region of the optic disk.

Early papilledema may not be symptomatic unless retinal hemorrhages or edema involve the macular area. Enlargement of the blind spot occurs after the ophthalmoscopic signs of papilledema occur (Table 7–1).

In patients with well-developed papilledema, there is transient obscuring of vision, unilateral or bilateral "blacking out" or "graying out" of vision, which can last for 15 seconds and can recur several times in a day. Later in the development of the disease, chronic papilledema occurs when there is associated secondary optic atrophy with subsequent severe visual loss. In chronic papilledema, there are irregular peripheral contraction and nerve fiber bundle defects in the visual field.

In papilledema, visual acuity is minimally decreased, visual field is normal, and pupillary reactions are normal. In papillitis, visual acuity, visual field, and pupillary reactions are abnormal.

Other signs and symptoms of papilledema are related to the increased intracranial pressure and the underlying central nervous system disorder: headache, nausea, vomiting, hemiparesis, hemianopias, and seizures.

Patients' Description of Symptoms

My vision became blurred for a few seconds; then it was okay.

Every so often, my vision blurs in the middle of the day.

I have the worst headache of my life, and I suddenly can't see very well—everything appears gray.

Examination and Management Summary

1. Perform the Snellen visual acuity assessment.

TABLE 7–1

MANAGEMENT OF THE SWOLLEN OPTIC DISK

1. Perform the Snellen visual acuity assessment.

2. Test for afferent pupillary defect. In papilledema, the pupillary reactions are normal.

3. Examine the optic nerve and macula.

4. Determine whether red desaturation is present.

5. Perform confrontation visual fields.

6. Check erythrocyte sedimentation rate.

7. If optic disk swelling is present, refer the patient to a neurologist or an ophthalmologist for further examination and evaluation.

2. Test for afferent pupillary defect. In papilledema, the pupillary reactions are normal.

3. Examine the optic nerve and macula with the direct hand-held ophthalmoscope.

4. If optic disk swelling is present, consider referring the patient to a neurologist for further examination and evaluation. If the optic nerve appears normal, consider referring the patient to an ophthalmologist.

PAPILLITIS

Papillitis is optic disk swelling caused by a local inflammatory process of the nerve head. Papillitis is usually acute and is almost always associated with moderate-to-severe vision loss—unilateral in adults and bilateral in children. However, in this entity, vision is moderately to severely decreased; the visual field demonstrates a centrocecal scotoma, and an afferent pupillary defect is present. Other features include the following: cells seen in the anterior vitreous near the optic nerve, loss of the central cup in the optic nerve, and deep retinal exudates in a star configuration in the macular region (Table 7–1).

In children, papillitis can be bilateral and is a common form of optic neuritis. It can be associated with viral illnesses, such as measles, mumps, and chickenpox. Tenderness of the globe and deep orbital pain may be present. Brow pain can be associated with eye movements. Most patients show an improvement of vision in the second or third week and may have normal vision by the fourth or fifth week. However, in some patients, recovery of vision may occur over several months. In a small number of cases, vision does not improve at all after the initial loss of vision.

Patients' Description of Symptoms

Suddenly I woke up, and I couldn't see out of my right eye.

My vision is strange; I don't see well out of one side of my eye.

Examination and Management Summary

1. Perform the Snellen visual acuity assessment: vision loss is at the 20/200 level.

2. Check for afferent pupillary defect, which is present in papillitis.

3. Visual field testing shows a centrocecal scotoma or a dark spot emanating from the optic nerve to central fixation. The dark spot can be elicited via confrontation visual field.

4. Refer the patient to a neurologist or an ophthalmologist for documentation, evaluation, and treatment.

5. Time to recovery of vision varies from 4 weeks to several months.

OPTIC NEURITIS

The term *optic neuritis* is usually reserved for primary inflammation of the nerve, including that occurring in demyelinating disease (Fig. 7–2; see also Fig. 7–2 Color Plate 10). Papillitis refers to the intraocular form of optic neuritis, in which optic disk swelling is variably affected. In adults, unilateral retrobulbar neuritis is common; in children, papillitis is the typical form of optic neuritis.

An associated viral illness involving the upper respiratory tract or gastrointestinal tract may be present. Coexisting neurologic signs and symptoms may be present, such as paresthesias, ataxia, diplopia, and sinus symptoms.

Patients usually have a moderate-to-severe visual loss, associated with pain in the orbit or globe area. Desaturation of colored objects; apparent reduction of light intensities; impairment of depth perception, especially with

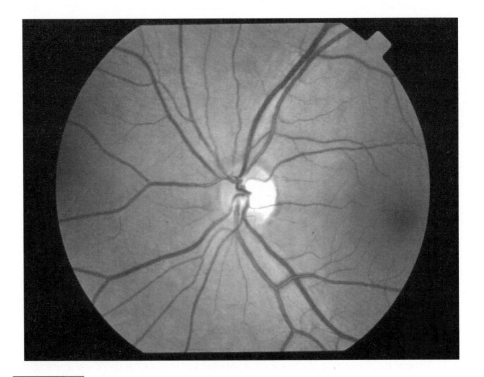

• **FIGURE 7–2**
Optic neuritis.

moving objects; and increase in visual deficit with exercise or elevation of body temperature occur (see Table 7–1).

The association of optic neuritis and demyelinating disease is common. Optic neuritis and internuclear ophthalmoplegia are the two most common ocular manifestations of multiple sclerosis.

In 1992, the Optic Neuritis Treatment Trial,[1] a multicenter, randomized clinical study, showed that visual function is recovered more quickly in patients treated with intravenous methylprednisolone than in the placebo group. The study, which involved 457 patients between the ages of 18 and 46 years, concluded that intravenous methylprednisolone followed by oral prednisone speeds the recovery of visual loss. Oral prednisone alone is an ineffective treatment and increases the risk of new episodes of optic neuritis.

Patients' Description of Symptoms

My eye hurts, and I cannot see.

The area around my eye hurts.

My favorite red dress looks discolored to me, yet my daughter says it looks the same.

I don't see colors very clearly now.

Examination and Management Summary

1. The patient may volunteer a history of a viral illness.

2. The Snellen visual acuity assessment shows loss of vision in one eye.

3. When the patient is tested with one eye closed, the color red appears normal yet the fellow eye sees the same color red as less red or desaturated.

4. On examination with a hand-held ophthalmoscope, the optic nerve shows some disk swelling or hyperemia.

5. Evaluation of the patient by a neurologist is helpful in making the diagnosis of optic neuritis and possible demyelinating disease.

6. Intravenous methylprednisolone followed by oral prednisone may be used in young to middle-aged patients with optic neuritis.

ANTERIOR ISCHEMIC OPTIC NEUROPATHY

Infarction of the anterior portion of the optic nerve that is unrelated to inflammation, demyelinization, or mass compression is poorly understood but common in the elderly population. It presents as unilateral disk swelling with severe visual loss.

Anterior ischemic optic neuropathy occurs in the sixth and seventh decade of life with altitudinal or other visual field defects involving central fixation. Subsequent improvement of vision is rare. The optic disk is swollen and has sector involvement and small flame hemorrhages (Table 7–1 and Fig. 7–3; see also Fig. 7–3 Color Plate 11). The swelling usually extends only a short distance beyond the border of the disk. Pain or other nonvisual symptoms are atypical. Optic atrophy ensues as disk edema resolves (Fig. 7–4; see also Fig. 7–4 Color Plate 11). The fellow eye is affected in 1/3 to 1/2 of patients. This disorder has no consistent relationship with hypertension, carotid atheromatous disease, or diabetes, nor is there evidence that any therapy in the form of corticosteroids, anticoagulants, or vasodilators alters the course of the disease in any way.

Patients' Description of Symptoms

I see a black spot when I read.

I am missing part of the television screen when I watch television.

I have a headache and blurred vision.

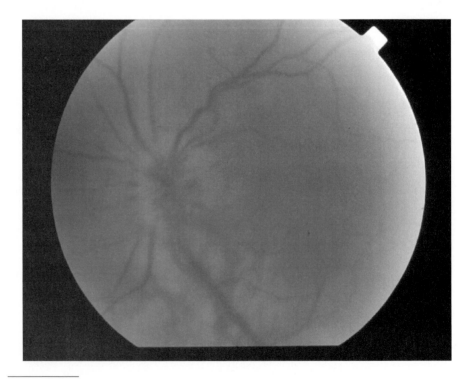

• **FIGURE 7–3**
Anterior ischemic optic neuropathy.

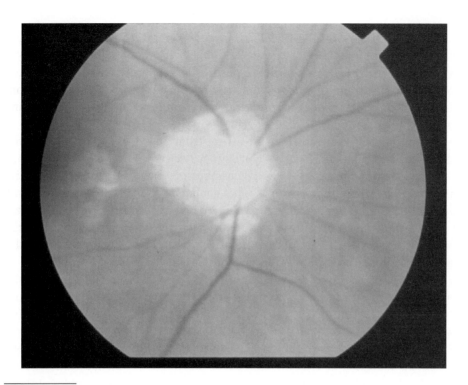

• **FIGURE 7–4**
Optic atrophy.

Examination and Management Summary

1. Perform the Snellen visual acuity assessment.

2. Perform confrontational visual field testing with the use of red objects. Look for the inability to see the intense color of red in one eye versus the other.

3. Look at the optic disk with the direct ophthalmoscope. Identify disk margins, pallor of disk, and optic disk edema.

4. If you have questions, refer the patient to a neurologist or an ophthalmologist.

TEMPORAL ARTERITIS

Temporal arteritis is a granulomatous inflammation of the intima of large or medium-sized arteries. It occurs in patients older than 60 years of age. It is slightly more common in women than in men and is rare in individuals of African and Asian descent. Systemic manifestations usually precede the clinical diagnosis by several months. The systemic symptoms include headaches, arthralgia, myalgia, fever, malaise, weight loss, anemia, and depression. Involvement of carotid, vertebral, basilar, or coronary arteries may produce central nervous system or cardiac disease, which can be fatal.

Facial artery involvement produces jaw claudication, tongue pain, and tongue infarction.

Dermatologic manifestations resulting from skin ischemia include vesicles, hemorrhagic bullae, focal skin crusting, necrosis, and ulceration.

The patient complains of a headache that is unabated, despite the use of aspirin or acetaminophen or rest. The headache may be described as one sided or bilateral. It may be accompanied by jaw pain or pain on mastication.

There may be only subtle visual loss in the beginning stages of the disease. However, with the complaints of jaw pain, headaches, or visual loss, the patient should be evaluated for temporal arteritis.

Polymyalgia rheumatica and cranial arteritis share some signs and symptoms, but they seem to be different diseases. Polymyalgia rheumatica occurs in patients older than 50 years, producing stiffness in the muscles of the neck, shoulders, upper arms, buttocks, and thighs. However, approximately 20% to 40% of patients with polymyalgia rheumatica also have cranial arteritis and are therefore at risk for blindness. Blindness is rare in patients with polymyalgia rheumatica who do not have the signs and symptoms of cranial arteritis.

Visual loss in temporal arteritis is due to an ischemic optic neuropathy. Optic nerve infarction is thought to arise from an involvement of the short posterior ciliary arteries. The disk is swollen and pale (Fig. 7–5; see also Fig. 7–5 Color Plate 11). Small hemorrhages surround the disk in the adjacent peripapillary retina. Cortical blindness resulting from occipital lobe infarction (blindness with normal fundus and no afferent pupillary defect), ischemic retinopathy (focal retinal ischemia with cotton wool spots), and retrobulbar ischemic optic neuropathy (vision loss, afferent pupillary defect, and normal fundus) are relatively rare causes of vision loss in cranial arteritis. Other central nervous system signs include cranial nerve palsies with associated cranial nerve palsies, ptosis, and miosis; these are thought to be due to ischemic necrosis of the extraocular muscles rather than of the ocular motor nerve.

Amaurosis fugax can occur in 2% to 19% of patients with cranial arteritis. Other unusual ocular signs and symptoms include visual hallucinations and orbital inflammatory pseudotumor.

The diagnosis is confirmed by an increased erythrocyte sedimentation rate. Although early in the disease process, the erythrocyte sedimentation rate may be normal. It usually ranges from 80 to 100 mm. It is important to make the diagnosis early because immediate administration of systemic corticosteroids produces dramatic improvement.

The disease activity is monitored by the erythrocyte sedimentation rate and the clinical state. The corticosteroid dose may have to be maintained for

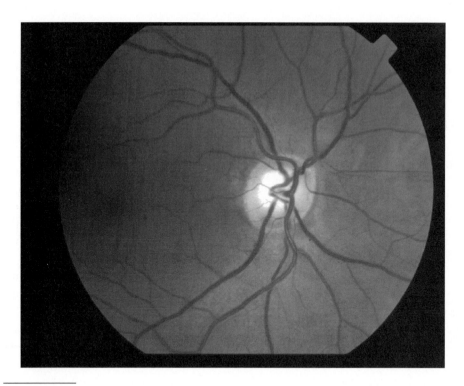

• **FIGURE 7–5**
Temporal arteritis.

several years and, if possible, with a maintenance dose of prednisolone below 5 mg.

Patients' Description of Symptoms

> I have pain when I chew.

> I haven't been able to see very well after my cataract surgery, and I have a constant headache.

> I have a dull aching headache, and I still can't see, even though I just got new glasses from my eye doctor.

Examination and Management Summary

1. Perform the Snellen visual acuity assessment.

2. The patient's pupillary examination is normal.

3. The hand-held ophthalmoscope shows a swollen and pale optic disk.

4. The patient may have a palpable temporal artery that is hard, enlarged, or engorged. The area may also be tender to palpation.

5. Check the erythrocyte sedimentation rate and refer the patient to an ophthalmologist or a surgeon for a temporal artery biopsy. Start prednisone therapy if the erythrocyte sedimentation rate is increased.

OTHER ABNORMALITIES OF THE OPTIC NERVE

Masquerade Syndromes

Visual loss from primary disease of the retina and optic nerve may be mistaken for central nervous system disease because they have a common ophthalmoscopic appearance. Patients in this category present with one or a combination of the following findings:

1. Elevation and enlargement of the optic nerve head.

2. Visual loss without fundus changes.

3. Optic atrophy.

PSEUDOPAPILLEDEMA OR OPTIC DISK EDEMA

Papilledema is defined as the blurring of optic disk margins caused by increased intracranial pressure, and the term *pseudopapilledema* is used to describe all of the causes of disk changes that may appear identical to, or be mistaken for, papilledema (Fig. 7–6; see also Fig. 7–6 Color Plate 11). Fluorescein angiography demonstrates capillary dilatation and permeability abnormalities of the juxtapapillary capillaries that extend beyond the edge of the optic disk swelling.

PSEUDOPAPILLEDEMA

Hyperopia

Patients with small eyes may have elevation of the optic nerve head by virtue of having a near-normal number of nerve fibers passing through a small optic nerve canal. Visual acuity is normal. Fluorescein angiography performed at the ophthalmologist's office can demonstrate absence of capillary dilatation existing beyond the optic disk margins.

Drusen of the Optic Disk

Patients with this disorder are usually asymptomatic or have an enlarged blind spot. Nodular deposits of extracellular material are located anterior to the lamina cribrosa, within the optic nerve head; they may be present at birth or may develop after birth (Figs. 7–7 and 7–8; see also Figs. 7–7 and 7–8, Color Plate 11).

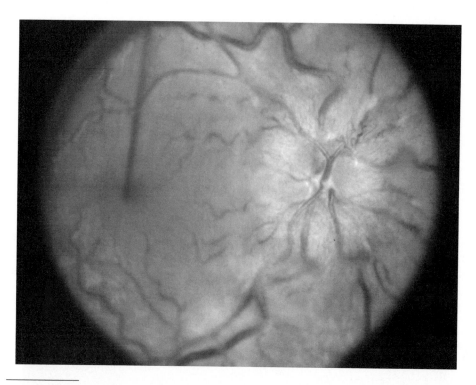

• **FIGURE 7–6**
Optic disk edema in Lyme disease.

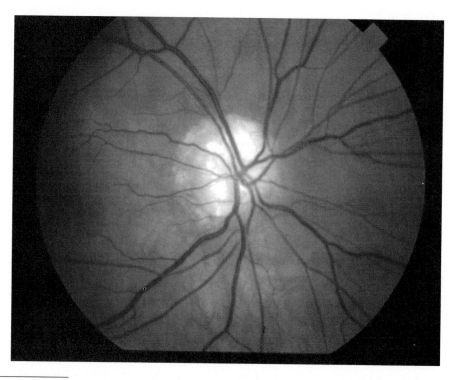

• **FIGURE 7–7**
Drusen of the optic nerve, showing nodular formation of the optic nerve head.

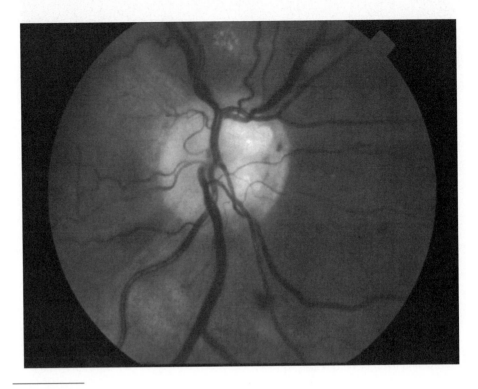

• **FIGURE 7–8**
Drusen of the optic nerve, showing displacement and gliosis of the overlying optic nerve vessels.

Malignant Hypertension

Patients with uncontrolled, severe hypertension may present with reduced visual acuity or transient obscurations of vision and show evidence of optic disk swelling in one or both eyes. Hemorrhages or exudates may be present (Fig. 7–9; see also Fig. 7–9 Color Plate 12).

Acute Disk Swelling in Insulin-Dependent Diabetes Mellitus

Patients with insulin-dependent diabetes mellitus may develop mild blurring of vision in one or both eyes, associated with disk swelling. This swelling is presumably related to a reversible vasculopathy because most patients show clearing of the edema and retain normal vision without requiring specific therapy.

Venous Stasis Papillopathy or Papillophlebitis

Patients with this condition are typically young or middle-aged adults who present with mild blurring of vision in one eye associated with swelling of the optic nerve head, mild venous engorgement, and a few retinal hemorrhages that are largely limited to the areas surrounding the optic disk. Visual

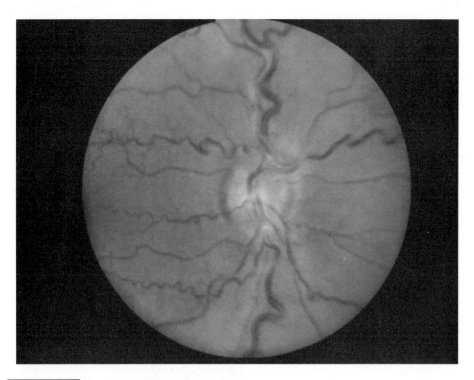

• **FIGURE 7–9**
Optic disk edema in malignant hypertension.

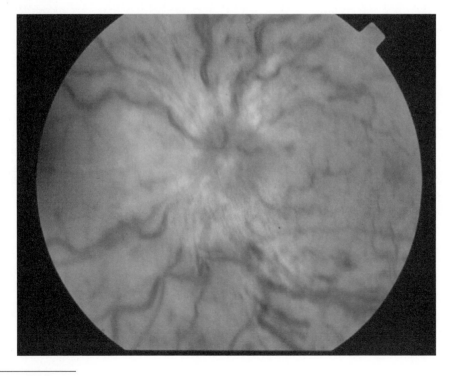

• **FIGURE 7–10**
Papillophlebitis.

field examination is characterized by an enlarged blind spot (Fig. 7–10; see also Fig. 7–10 Color Plate 12). Most patients experience spontaneous recovery without any treatment, and the fundus usually returns to normal.

Reference

1. Beck RM, Cleary PA, Anderson MA: Randomized controlled trial of corticosteroids in the treatment of acute optic neuritis. N Engl J Med 326:581–588, 1992.

8

Primary Tumors of the Eye

Primary tumors of the eye are rare. Early diagnosis of these growths is possible because tumors are usually visible, displacing the eyeball and affecting vision adversely. The hallmark of malignancy is its asymmetry and rapid rate of growth, associated with loss of function. For example, in rhabdomyosarcoma, the most common malignant orbital tumor of mesenchymal origin in the orbit, there is orbital proptosis, rapid loss of vision, and accompanying pain from the mass effect of the orbit pressing against its contents (Fig. 8–1). The entities discussed in this chapter necessitate prompt referral to an ophthalmologist. The recognition of these ocular entities is important in the management of the patient in a primary care setting (Table 8–1).

PRIMARY MALIGNANT TUMORS OF THE EYELIDS

Basal cell carcinoma is the most common eyelid carcinoma. It affects individuals older than 50 years and is related to sun exposure. Usually, it is seen in the margin of the lower eyelid or orbital area (Fig. 8–2; see also Fig. 3–18). Basal cell carcinoma is slow growing and locally invasive and does not spread to the regional lymph nodes.

Basal cell carcinoma begins like a small ulcer with an irregular nodular border and indurated base. Small clusters of basal cell carcinoma may grow near the eyelids and orbit; these clusters can be seen with a magnifying glass. The basal cell carcinoma can also present as a large rodent ulcer, 4 to 5 mm in diameter.

Basal carcinoma found on the lower eyelid but close to the medial canthus invades the structures of the medial canthus and the orbit. These cases require complete eradication. The sclerosing or morphea-like basal cell carcinoma can present after delayed diagnosis because it lies beneath the skin

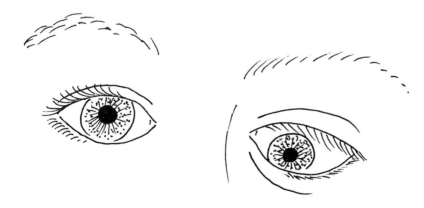

• **FIGURE 8–1**
Rhabdomyosarcoma.

TABLE 8–1

TUMOR DIAGNOSIS

1. Perform the Snellen visual acuity assessment.

2. Perform a penlight examination of the eyelids, orbit, and external anatomy of the globe.

3. Look for asymmetry, ectropion, entropion, proptosis, discoloration, and hyperpigmentation.

4. Look at the extraocular movement: is there asymmetry?

5. Record the dimensions of the area of growth. Take a Polaroid photograph of the area or make a sketch of the lesion on the examination note.

6. Refer the patient to an ophthalmologist.

surface and manifests as alopecia, eyelid notching, ectropion (eyelid eversion), or entropion (eyelid inversion).

Squamous cell carcinoma grows slowly and painlessly for many months before it is noticed. It is locally aggressive, spreading to the lymphatic system, surrounding skin, connective tissue, cartilage, and bone. In the late stages, there is severe pain.

Squamous cell carcinoma begins as a small wartlike growth with keratotic covering, then becoming an ulcer with local induration and hyperemia (Fig. 8–3).

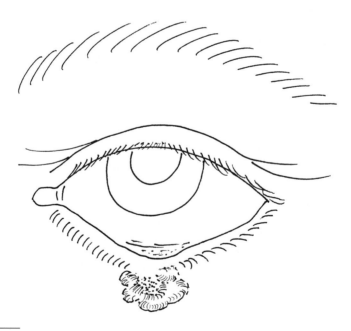

• **FIGURE 8–2**
Basal cell carcinoma of the lower eyelid with associated ectropion.

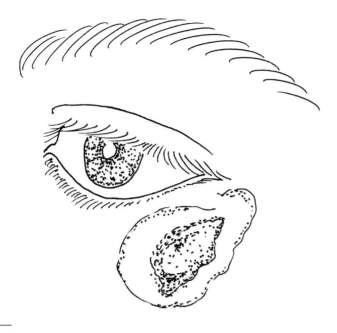

- **FIGURE 8–3**
Squamous cell carcinoma.

Sebaceous gland carcinomas, arising from the glands of Zeis or meibomian glands of the eyelids can present as chronic blepharitis, conjunctivitis, or chalazion (stye). These tumors are aggressive and require referral to the ophthalmologist.

Excision of these malignant growths is the procedure of choice. Frozen sections are used to ensure complete excision and skin margins free of tumor.

Patients' Description of Symptoms

I have a growth on my eyelid. It doesn't really bother me, but it's bleeding now.

I have had a red itchy eye for 6 months, and all the drops and ointments you gave me haven't worked. It's still bothering me.

My eyelid is turning out on one side.

Examination and Management Summary

1. Perform the Snellen visual acuity assessment.

2. Examine the area of abnormal growth. Take a Polaroid photograph of the area, or draw and label its dimensions on the examination note.

3. Refer the patient to an ophthalmologist.

PRIMARY MALIGNANT TUMOR OF THE CONJUNCTIVA

Lymphoma is uncommon but can appear spontaneously in adults or as part of systemic lymphosarcoma, lymphocytic leukemia, Hodgkin's disease, or related conditions (see Fig. 3–20). Biopsy is important for establishing the diagnosis, and radiotherapy is the treatment of choice.

Squamous cell carcinoma is rare but presents in the conjunctiva as a white lesion with raised borders and sometimes deposits of heaped up collagenous growth.

Melanoma of the conjunctiva is also rare but presents as aggressive pigment growth over weeks or months (Fig. 8–4; see also Fig. 8–4 Color Plate 12). The pigmentation has irregular edges and has areas of darker pigmentation associated with areas of lighter pigmentation. There can be associated bleeding.

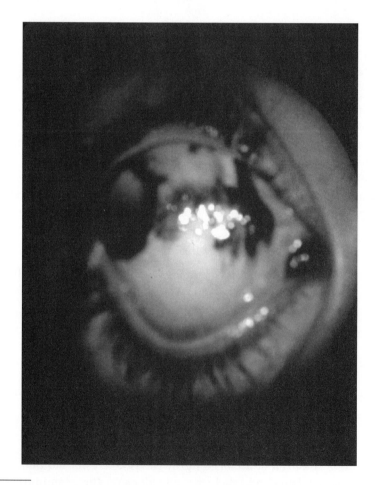

• **FIGURE 8–4**
Melanoma of the conjunctiva.

Patients' Description of Symptoms

The brown spot on my eye has changed color from brown to black in one month.

I scratched a pimple on my eyelid, and now it's gotten bigger and hard.

My eyelid won't close right and feels hard when I touch it. I have pain in that area.

Examination and Management Summary

1. Perform the Snellen visual acuity assessment.

2. Photograph the area of growth or draw and label its dimensions on the examination note.

3. Refer the patient to an ophthalmologist.

PRIMARY MALIGNANT ORBITAL TUMORS

Rhabdomyosarcoma is the most common orbital malignancy of mesenchymal origin in the orbit (see Fig. 8–1). This tumor is most frequently found in Caucasians younger than 10 years and has a slight male preponderance. There is usually proptosis downward and temporally as well as rapid growth. Metastases to the brain and lungs are common. Irradiation has improved the prognosis of this highly malignant tumor. Exenteration is necessary in some cases.

Patients' Description of Symptoms

My son's eye bulged out in the past 2 weeks. We thought it was related to a fall, but we are worried.

My child woke up one day with his eye slightly red, and over the next few days, his eyelids wouldn't close over the eye.

Examination and Management Summary

1. Perform the Snellen visual acuity assessment. The results may be very poor.

2. Note the area of asymmetry. Note the proptosis. Photograph or sketch the lesion. Note the displacement of the adjacent anatomy.

3. Refer the patient to an ophthalmologist.

PRIMARY MALIGNANT TUMORS OF THE RETINA AND CHOROID

Retinoblastoma in children is a rare but life-threatening tumor of childhood (Fig. 8–5; see also Fig. 8–5 Color Plate 12). Ninety percent of cases appear before the end of the fifth year of life. It is bilateral in 30% of cases. Retinoblastoma occurs in 1/18,000 live births, or in 11 cases per one million children younger than 5 years. Retinoblastoma arises as a large, nodular, whitish tumor in the posterior retina.

Retinoblastoma usually remains unnoticed until it has advanced far enough to produce a white pupil (leukokoria) (Fig. 8–6; see also Fig. 8–6 Color Plate 12) or strabismus, noticed by a family member or a primary care physician. Strabismus is the initial symptom in one of every five patients with retinoblastoma. Other signs and symptoms are red, painful eye with glaucoma, poor vision, and an orbital cellulitis–like condition.

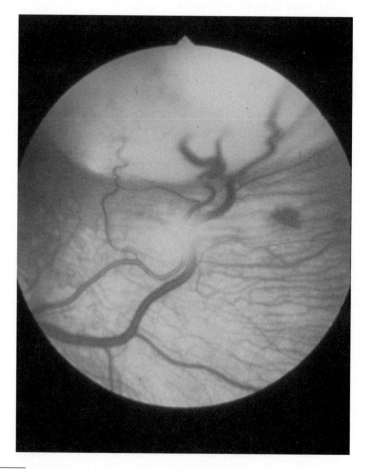

• **FIGURE 8–5**
Retinoblastoma.

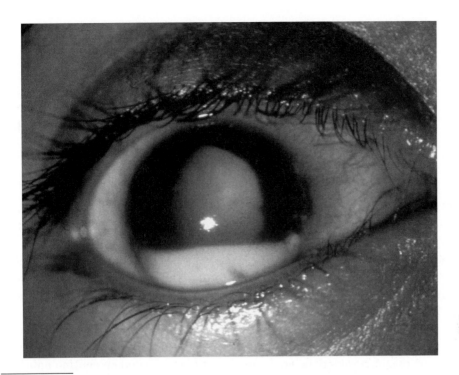

• FIGURE 8–6
Leukokoria (white reflex) and hypopyon in a child with retinoblastoma.

The retinoblastoma locus in the 13q14 is the physical location of a large gene that codes for a 4.73 kilomessage. An intact gene appears to protect against malignancy. Both copies of the gene at the retinoblastoma locus must be destroyed, lost, mutated, or inactivated for retinoblastoma to be initiated.

About 94% of retinoblastomas arise by mutation; therefore, only 6% are familial. When familial inheritance is suspected, a retinoblastoma survivor has an approximately 50% chance of producing an affected child.

Enucleation is the treatment of choice for large tumors. Radiation or chemotherapy is used in the treatment of bilateral tumors.

Patients' Description of Symptoms

I saw a recent photo of my baby with my family. Everyone has a red eye with the flash except my baby—one of his eyes has a white growth over it.

My child's eyes are turning in.

My daughter has a white growth over her eye.

My son keeps rubbing one eye, over and over.

Examination and Management Summary

1. In infants and toddlers, visual acuity may be difficult to ascertain.

2. Look at the eye in question. Is the eye turning in or turning out?

3. Is there a white reflex? Examine the young patient with a flashlight.

4. Refer the patient to an ophthalmologist.

MALIGNANT MELANOMA OF THE CHOROID

Choroidal melanoma is the most common primary intraocular malignancy. It is the main primary intraocular disease that can be fatal in adults. The disease is most often diagnosed in the sixth decade of life. It is slightly more common in males. Approximately six cases of choroidal melanoma exist per million per year.

The chief complaint of the patient is usually a loss of vision that results from an associated retinal detachment, a large tumor growth near the optic nerve or macular region, or an asymptomatic lesion seen on routine ophthalmic evaluation.

For primary care specialists, the diagnosis is difficult unless the patient specifically complains of visual loss. In examining the patient with a direct, hand-held ophthalmoscope, the physician can ascertain the loss of the red reflex, and in its place, a white reflex may be present. This phenomenon suggests the presence of a serious eye disorder, which necessitates a referral to the ophthalmologist.

Most patients with choroidal melanoma present with retinal detachment. The typical presentation is a pigmented collar-button–shaped tumor, usually associated with an overlying exudative retinal detachment (Fig. 8–7; see also Fig. 8–7 Color Plate 12). By this time, the patient usually has profound visual loss in the affected eye.

The tumor is classified according to six cell types of the Callender classification: spindle A, spindle B, fascicular, epithelioid, mixed, and necrotic. The epithelioid, mixed, and necrotic cell types carry the worst prognosis for survival. Other prognostic factors include extrascleral extension, tumor size, and tumor location.

Systemic evaluation is directed at frequent sites of metastatic involvement: liver, lung, bone, and subcutaneous tissues. Examination should include complete physical examination with attention to the skin and subcutaneous tissues, routine chest x-ray and serum liver function studies (serum gamma-glutamyl transpeptidase, serum lactic dehydrogenase, and aspartate transaminase levels). If the liver function results are abnormal, ultrasonography or computed tomography of the liver should be performed. Routine brain or hepatic imaging studies are not recommended.

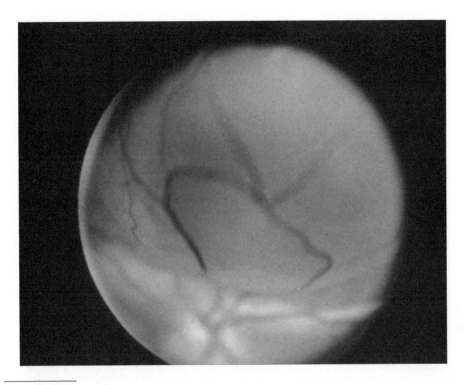

• **FIGURE 8–7**
Malignant melanoma of the choroid.

Depending on the size of the tumor, periodic observation can be performed at the ophthalmologist's office. Photocoagulation is a viable treatment modality for selected tumors that are less than 3 mm in diameter and are located more than 3 mm from the fovea. Radiotherapy is widely used for posterior uveal melanomas. The most commonly used isotopes are cobalt 60, ruthenium 106, iridium 192, and iodine 125. The decision regarding the type of plaque chosen is usually coordinated with the radiation oncologist. Proton-beam irradiation is also used for treatment. The type of radiotherapy available varies according to different ocular oncology centers. Enucleation is the traditional treatment, especially in cases in which an advanced tumor occupies most of the intraocular structure and produces secondary glaucoma. Orbital exenteration is used in the rare instances of massive orbital extension in a blind, uncomfortable eye and in primary orbital extension.

Patients' Description of Symptoms

I can't see out of my left eye.

I could never see well after cataract surgery.

The whites of my eyes turned color.

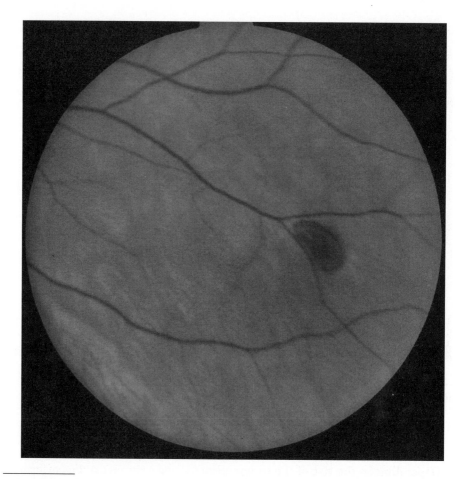

• **FIGURE 8–8**
Choroidal nevus, which can be confused with malignant melanoma of the choroid.

Examination and Management Summary

1. Perform the Snellen visual acuity assessment; the results may be very poor.

2. Use the hand-held direct ophthalmoscope to look inside the retina. If white reflex or derangement of retinal architecture is seen, refer the patient to an ophthalmologist.

3. If a small, flat, pigmented lesion is present, it may be a nevus (Fig. 8–8; see also Fig. 8–8 Color Plate 12). Refer the patient to an ophthalmologist for confirmation.

9

Examination of the Pediatric Patient

EMBRYOLOGY

Some of the eye problems of the newborn are related to the embryologic proximity of various structures within the eye at approximately the fifth week of life. The lens is originally next to a mesenchyme that becomes the vitreous and the pupil. Thus, there are abnormalities of the lens, vitreous, and retina that have their origins in the improper development of the eye at this stage.

SPECIAL EXAMINATION TECHNIQUES (Table 9–1)

The most important element of the examination of an infant or child is gentleness. The child should be as relaxed as possible. The primary care physician may ask the mother to hold the child as the examination begins. The physician may use toys to distract the young child during the examination.

If possible, the examination should be made into a game. The child can be provided with a puppet who is holding a small visual acuity chart or calibrated E cards (see Appendix for a listing of companies that manufacture these items) (Fig. 9–1). The physician may use the swinging flashlight in one hand and hold a toy over it so that the child looks at the light and the toy at the same time (Fig. 9–2). The patient should be rewarded with stickers or lollipops after the examination—the accompanying parent will be grateful to the physician.

For the young patient, it is important to ascertain if he or she can see. In preverbal children, the use of an optokinetic tape (Fig. 9–3) can elicit a characteristic optokinetic nystagmus, indicating that the child can fix and

---

TABLE 9–1

THE PEDIATRIC EXAMINATION

Infants
    Use the penlight to ascertain if the infant can fixate and follow the light. Otherwise, refer the infant to an ophthalmologist.
Preverbal children
    Perform a penlight examination of the pupils and observe the extraocular movements. A toy puppet is a good fixation device for this age group.
Nursery school–aged children
    Try using an E chart devised for children.
    If this is unsuccessful, use the preverbal children methods listed above.
School-aged children
    Test visual acuity with the Snellen eye chart.
All children
    Test with one eye covered at a time. Each eye may respond differently, suggesting asymmetric visual potential. Note if an infant shows a preference for one eye and tell the ophthalmologist.
If you have any questions, refer the child to an ophthalmologist.

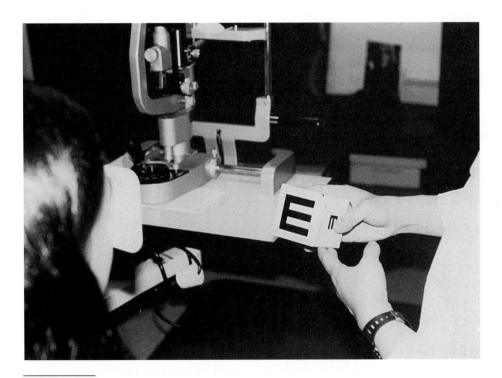

• **FIGURE 9–1**
E-block.

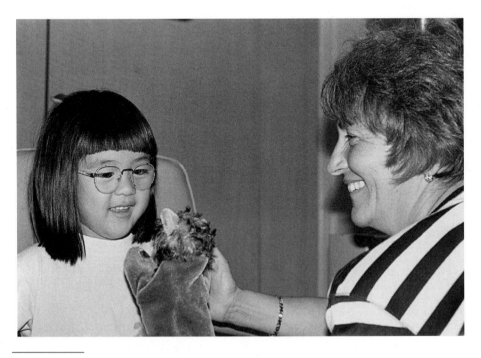

• **FIGURE 9–2**
Physician using toy as a fixation device for purposes of examination. Photography by Irwin Sterbakov.

162

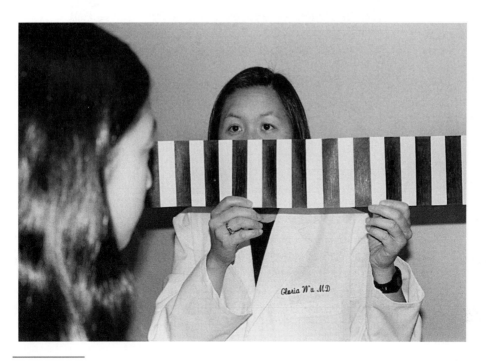

• **FIGURE 9–3**
Optokinetic tape. Photography by Irwin Sterbakov.

follow at a 20/200 vision level. Toddlers or nursery school–aged children can read the special visual acuity chart with animal diagrams calibrated to the 20/30 level, approximating the Snellen visual acuity chart. In the school-aged child who knows the alphabet, the regular Snellen chart is adequate.

Examination of the Newborn

The normal eye in infants may be small, with a slight epicanthal fold, called *pseudoepicanthus* (Fig. 9–4). This change in the lid fold is gradually lengthened as the face gets larger and fuller with growth and development.

A few upward-pointing eyelashes from the lower eyelid may be present in the medial canthus. Unless eye irritation is present, this condition does not require treatment and resolves as the eye grows and lengthens. In cases of eye irritation caused by the misdirection of the eyelashes, the primary care physician can refer the patient to an ophthalmologist.

Shortly after birth, the newborn may have a discharge from the eye. This may be due to an immature tear duct system; ocular massage at that tear duct opening is helpful (Fig. 9–5). Referral to the ophthalmologist may be helpful if the discharge is persistent after a few weeks.

At birth, the newborn may have a discharge, commonly called *ophthalmia neonatorum*.

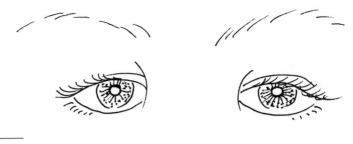

• **FIGURE 9–4**
Epicanthus.

Congenital ptosis may be present such that one eyelid is slightly lower on the patient's pupil on one side (Fig. 9–6). If the eyelid does not elevate at all on one side, the patient receives no light stimulation from that one side, and consequently, the associated visual cortex is undeveloped as well. In these cases, immediate referral to an ophthalmologist for evaluation and possible ptosis surgery may help the patient attain his or her full potential for vision.

Examination of the Premature Infant

The premature infant may have a host of abnormalities associated with the visual pathways. Of paramount concern is the diagnosis of the entity *retinopathy of prematurity*, in which the patient can have abnormal blood vessel growth with concomitant bleeding and retinal detachment (Figs. 9–7 and 9–8). The risk factors for retinopathy of prematurity are low birth weight, history of intrauterine infections, fetal alcohol syndrome, hydrocephalus, intrauterine growth retardation, and duration and concentration of oxygen exposure in the prenatal period. Although it is now thought that low birth

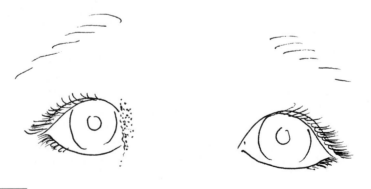

• **FIGURE 9–5**
Blocked tear duct in an infant.

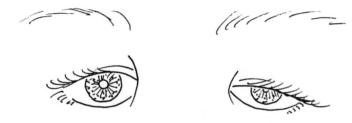

• **FIGURE 9–6**
Congenital ptosis.

weight is the most significant risk factor, it is not clear as to why only 5% to 10% of low-birth-weight babies have retinopathy of prematurity. Much more research is being conducted to understand more fully the pathogenesis of this entity.

The examination of the newborn requires the use of the direct ophthalmoscope to identify any abnormalities of the eye. Bleeding may occur in the anterior chamber or the folds in the cornea as a result of forceps or traumatic delivery. The patient may need examination by a specialist in pediatric oph-

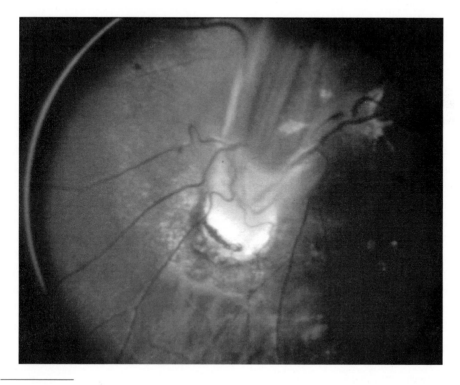

• **FIGURE 9–7**
Retinopathy of prematurity, dragged optic disk.

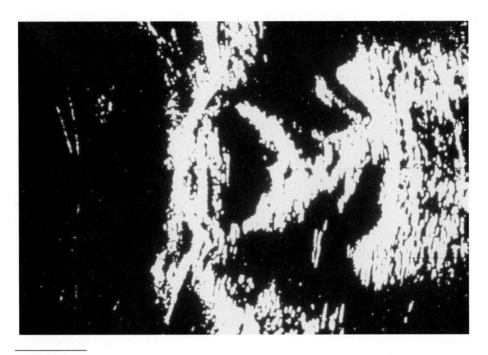

• **FIGURE 9–8**
Ultrasound of retinal detachment in retinopathy of prematurity.

thalmology. In some cases, examination under anesthesia is necessary in these newborn infants.

STRABISMUS

The child may present with crossed eyes or widely diverging eyes at a distance or near (Fig. 9–9). The child may have a parent who had a similar problem as a child but had successful surgery. Although some instances are obvious on physical examination, others require an ophthalmic consultation.

Snellen visual acuity assessment is useful in the verbal child, but in the preverbal child, the diagnosis may be a challenge. Special testing at an ophthalmologist's office may be necessary.

Although the subtle forms of strabismus are hard to see in a primary care setting, the physician should notice that the vision is asymmetric. The affected eye sees less well than the other eye. If both eyes cross or diverge, the patient has a dominant, fixating eye that has relatively better vision than the other eye.

Patients' Description of Symptoms

My child's eyes cross when he is tired.

My daughter's right eye wanders.

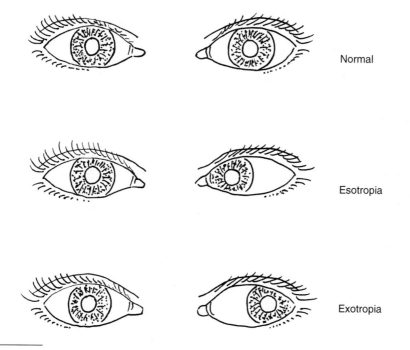

Normal

Esotropia

Exotropia

• **FIGURE 9–9**
Strabismus.

My son twists his head when he looks at signs in the distance.

My son's eyes look crossed sometimes, then straight at other times.

My daughter's eyes don't move together.

Examination and Management Summary

1. Testing visual acuity is difficult in children until they are of school age.
   a. *Infants and toddlers*: test their pupillary light reflexes and watch to see whether they can fixate and follow the penlight as you move it to test cranial nerves III, IV, and VI (the medial rectus muscle moves the eye medially, the superior and inferior rectus muscles move the eyes vertically, and the lateral rectus muscle moves the eye laterally).
   b. *Nursery school–aged children*: test as you would infants and toddlers, and also test their visual acuity with the eye chart. Specialized children's eye charts are available (see Appendix).
   c. *School-aged children*: test visual acuity with the Snellen eye chart.

2. Do the eyes cross inward or diverge when the child is looking straight ahead at a distant object?

3. Hold up an object in close proximity to the child: do the child's eyes cross or diverge when he or she is looking at the near object?

4. If you have any questions, refer the patient to an ophthalmologist.

AMBLYOPIA, OR "LAZY EYE"

Amblyopia occurs when the eye, although anatomically normal, does not see the 20/20 line on the Snellen acuity chart. This can occur if the child did not receive proper corrective glasses at an early enough age. It is postulated that the brain's visual cortex and the eye do not develop at the same rate if the eye does not receive clear, focused vision in the formative years of the first decade of life.

Patients often say that one eye has had poor vision as long as they can remember. As a child, the patient may not have been seen by an ophthalmologist and never received corrective lenses. Perhaps one eye was very near-sighted or farsighted, so that it never sent messages to the visual cortex, resulting in loss of vision. With sophisticated visual electrophysiology, abnormalities may be detected, even when the eye appears anatomically normal.

The child may never realize that one eye sees better than the other until one eye is accidentally covered in play activities. In a preverbal child, the mother may notice that the child favors one side over the other. Thus, it is important for all children to be examined by an ophthalmologist to ascertain their visual potential in each eye.

Patients' Description of Symptoms

I can't see when I cover my right eye.

My child turns his head to one side to watch television.

I've seen my daughter walk into walls.

My child walks into objects all the time.

My son holds his head so close to the books that he is reading.

Examination and Management Summary

1. Testing visual acuity is difficult in children until they are of school age.
   a. *Infants and toddlers*: test their pupillary light reflexes and watch to see whether they can fixate and follow the penlight as you move it to test cranial nerves III, IV, and VI (the medial rectus muscle moves the eye medially, the superior and inferior rectus muscles move the eyes vertically, and the lateral rectus muscle moves the eye laterally).

    b. *Nursery school–aged children*: test as you would infants and toddlers, and also test their visual acuity with the eye chart. Specialized children's eye charts are available (see Appendix).

    c. *School-aged children*: test visual acuity with the Snellen eye chart.

2. Test all the children with one of their eyes covered at a time. Each eye may have a different response, suggesting asymmetric visual potential. Infants may show preferential looking out of one eye. This phenomenon should be noted and reported to an ophthalmologist.

3. If you have any questions, refer the child to an ophthalmologist.

10

Ophthalmic Emergencies

CHIEF COMPLAINT AND THE HISTORY OF THE PRESENT ILLNESS

The most important chief complaint in ophthalmic emergencies is loss of vision. The second most important chief complaint is loss of vision with pain. These two symptoms alert the practitioner that the patient is experiencing an emergency (Table 10–1).

The next questions the patient should be asked are

1. Is the visual loss transient, lasting only minutes, or has the loss of vision persisted for days?

2. Is there associated pain? Has there been trauma associated with this symptom? Is there severe pain, with visual loss associated with nausea and vomiting? This is the hallmark symptom complex of acute angle closure glaucoma.

REVIEW OF SYSTEMS AS IT RELATES TO OPHTHALMOLOGY

1. Is there prior history of glaucoma in the patient or in family members? Has anyone else in the family had an acute glaucoma attack requiring immediate care?

2. Is there a history of vascular ischemia? This is important for retinal vein occlusion or artery occlusion, which can cause sudden loss of vision.

3. Is there a history of retinal detachment or retinal disease? For patients experiencing floaters and flashes of light, retinal detachment is a prime consideration.

4. Is there a history of thyroid disease? People with dry eye have a tendency toward corneal abrasions with contact lens use.
5. Systemic disease.
   a. *Diabetes.* The longer the duration of the disease, the more likely it is that diabetic retinopathy is present in the patient. Patients with insulin-dependent (type I) diabetes mellitus may have a higher

---

TABLE 10–1

REASONS FOR IMMEDIATE REFERRAL TO AN OPHTHALMOLOGIST

1. Severe eye pain.

2. Loss of vision, sudden or gradual.

3. Eye trauma.

frequency of diabetic retinopathy, but patients with non–insulin-dependent (type II) diabetes mellitus have mild symptoms of visual loss that may be ignored by the patient until it is very late in the course of the disease process.

b. *Hypertension.* Patients who have uncontrolled or poorly controlled hypertension are at risk for retinal strokes and vascular occlusive disease. All the entities can cause transient visual loss.

c. *Coronary artery disease.* Patients who have had coronary artery bypass grafting are predisposed to vascular occlusive disease of the retina. In addition, these patients have a history of vascular ischemia, which may have far-reaching physiologic consequences.

d. *Cancer.* Lung cancer, breast cancer, and colon cancer can manifest as metastatic lesions in the eye.

Examination Summary (see Chapter 2)

1. Perform the Snellen visual acuity assessment.

2. Perform a pupillary evaluation.

3. Perform a penlight examination.

4. Evaluate the optic nerve, retina, and macula with the hand-held direct ophthalmoscope.

EYE PAIN

Eye Pain Related to Minor Trauma

Although the pain resulting from corneal abrasions can be excruciating, there is no real loss of vision and no headache or nausea. The patient usually explains that he or she scratched the cornea or that the pain is related to contact lens overwear.

Summary of Clinical Presentation

1. Eye pain associated with scratch to the cornea.

2. Discomfort ranging from mild to severe.

3. Retention of good visual acuity.

Examination and Management Summary

1. Use the penlight with a fluorescein strip to ascertain the abrasion.

2. Use antibiotic ophthalmic ointment and patch the eye closed for 24 hours. Refer the patient to an ophthalmologist for further evaluation.

SUDDEN LOSS OF VISION

Sudden loss of vision may mean that the patient is experiencing a partial or complete retinal vascular occlusion. The partial vascular insults are branch retinal vein occlusion or branch retinal artery occlusion. Complete vascular occlusion of the eye can manifest as central retinal vein occlusion and central retinal artery occlusion. The other possibilities include a retinal detachment, which can occur in both the young and the elderly. The symptoms are sudden loss of vision associated with floaters or photopsia ("flashing lights").

Myopes or contact lens wearers are more prone to this condition.

Summary of Clinical Presentation

1. Loss of vision.

2. Absence of pain.

3. Absence of redness of the eyes.

Examination and Management Summary

1. Using the direct ophthalmoscope, look for hemorrhages along the retinal vessels, which can occur with retinal vein occlusion.

2. If a white or dull macular or retinal reflex is found instead of a red reflex, a retinal artery occlusion may be present.

3. In a retinal detachment, the direct ophthalmoscope reveals a whitish ballooning retina instead of the usual orange-red reflex of the eye.

4. Refer the patient to an ophthalmologist immediately.

EYE PAIN AND SUDDEN LOSS OF VISION

When the patient has severe pain in the eye, it is important to consider a diagnosis of angle closure glaucoma. The patient's complaint usually is, "This is the worst pain that I have ever had in my eye, and I feel sick to my stomach."

Summary of Clinical Presentation

1. Eye pain.

2. Red eye.

3. Sudden loss of vision.

4. Nausea and/or headache.

Examination and Management Summary

1. Refer the patient immediately to an ophthalmologist.

2. If no ophthalmologist is available, immediately begin administering acetazolamide, 500 mg sequels orally every 12 hours, until an ophthalmologist can be reached.

TRAUMA TO THE EYE

If the patient has a history of blunt trauma to the eye or the orbit, he or she should be referred to an ophthalmologist immediately. If no ophthalmologist is available, the patient should be made comfortable, and the eye should not be forced open for examination purposes.

Examination and Management Summary

1. If the patient presents with a hemorrhagic, swollen eye after blunt trauma, do not force open the eye. There may be serious damage that may require examination in the operating room, with the patient under anesthesia.

2. If the patient presents with a red eye, but the eye is open, and the eyelids appear hemorrhagic, test the patient in the usual manner:
   a. Snellen visual acuity.
   b. Penlight examination.
   c. Direct ophthalmoscope examination.

3. Call an ophthalmologist for further direction, or refer the patient to the ophthalmologist's office. Sometimes, even though the visual acuity may be preserved, there may be serious problems inside the eye that only the ophthalmologist can determine.

4. Administer tetanus toxoid to the patient if he or she has a penetrating injury.

5. Put a plastic or metal eye shield over the eye as the patient is awaiting transport.

Appendix

Appendix

COMMONLY USED EYE MEDICATIONS

A. Antibiotics.
   1. Ointments (most are for gram-positive coverage).
      a. *Erythromycin ophthalmic ointment*: least irritating to the cornea.
      b. *Bacitracin ophthalmic ointment*: commonly used.
      c. *Polymyxin B sulfate–bacitracin zinc (Polysporin) ophthalmic ointment*: can cause redness and dryness of the eyes.
      d. *Tetracycline ophthalmic ointment*: hard to find in pharmacies; used for acne rosacea and for patients allergic to aforementioned antibiotic ointments.
   2. Eyedrops.
      a. *Gentamicin, tobramycin*: can be irritating to the cornea but excellent for postoperative and other minor infections. Provide gram-negative coverage.
      b. *Sulfacetamide*: has been used for mild conjunctivitis but has been known to rarely cause Stevens-Johnson syndrome. Provides gram-negative coverage.
      c. *Ciprofloxacin hydrochloride (HCl)*: provides broad-spectrum coverage for gram-negative and gram-positive organisms.
      d. *Ofloxacin 0.3%*: provides broad-spectrum coverage for gram-negative and gram-positive organisms.
B. Steroids (eyedrops). Steroids can cause transient intraocular pressure elevation and glaucoma.
   1. *Prednisolone acetate 1/8%*: used for maintenance treatment for herpetic eye conditions and chronic uveitis of the eye, or for long-term postoperative management of corneal graft rejection.
   2. *Prednisolone acetate 1%*: standard treatment for inflammatory conditions of the eye.
   3. *Fluorometholone*: has fewer intraocular pressure effects.
   4. *Rimexolone*: has anti-inflammatory effects but does not affect intraocular pressure.
C. Nonsteroidal anti-inflammatory agents (eyedrops): prostaglandins have been shown in animal models to be mediators of certain kinds of intraocular inflammation. These nonsteroidal anti-inflammatory agents act on various steps of prostaglandin synthesis.
   1. *Flurbiprofen sodium 0.03%*: inhibits cyclo-oxygenase, which is needed for the synthesis of prostaglandin.
   2. *Diclofenac sodium 0.1%*: inhibits cyclo-oxygenase, which is necessary in prostaglandin synthesis.
D. Antiglaucoma medications.
   1. Ointments.
      a. *Pilopine HS gel (pilocarpine in ointment form)*: see below.

2. Eyedrops.
   a. Parasympathomimetic agents:
      Miotics: increase aqueous outflow facility.
      (1) *Pilocarpine 0.5%, 1%, 2%, 3%, 4%, 6%*: systemic side effects include diaphoresis (perspiration); stimulation of glands, including salivary, lacrimal, gastric, and respiratory mucosa. Contraction of smooth muscle involving the gastrointestinal tract may lead to diarrhea, nausea, abdominal cramps, and malaise. Blood pressure may rise or fall, depending on the degree of autonomic stimulation. High concentrations of pilocarpine may weaken myocardial contractility.
      (2) *Carbachol 1.5%, 3%*: systemic side effects are similar to those of pilocarpine, noted earlier.
      (3) *Echothiophate 0.06%, 0.125%, 0.25%*: inhibitor of acetylcholinesterase. Systemic side effects are related to cholinesterase depletion. Echothiophate iodide depletes both true cholinesterase in red blood cells and pseudocholinesterase in plasma. Pseudocholinesterase hydrolyzes succinylcholine. General anesthesia may lead to prolonged respiratory paralysis in patients using echothiophate iodide. Echothiophate iodide may cause parasympathomimetic reactions, such as diarrhea, nausea, abdominal cramps, and malaise. The antidote for echothiophate iodide toxicity is pralidoxime chloride (Protopam), which frees cholinesterase from the complex and prevents further inhibition but does not alter the intraocular pressure–lowering effect.
   b. Adrenergic agonists: decrease aqueous production:
      (1) *Epinephrine HCl 0.5%, 1%, 2%*
      (2) *Dipivalyl epinephrine 0.1%*: this compound is hydrolyzed to epinephrine after it is absorbed into the eye. Systemic side effects include elevated blood pressure, tachycardia, arrhythmias, headache, and anxiety.
   c. Beta-adrenergic antagonists:
      (1) *Timolol maleate 0.25%, 0.5%*: timolol maleate is a beta$_1$- and beta$_2$-adrenergic antagonist, which works by reducing aqueous production. It is contraindicated in patients with asthma. Timolol maleate has systemic side effects related to its systemic blockade of beta$_1$-adrenergic receptors, leading to cardiovascular changes such as bradycardia, arrhythmias, heart failure, and syncope. It has respiratory effects caused by its blockade of beta$_2$-adrenergic receptors, leading to bronchospasm and airway obstruction in asthmatics. Central nervous system effects include depression, fatigue, sexual impotence, and emotional lability.
      (2) *Betaxolol HCl 0.25%, 0.5%*: a beta$_1$-adrenergic, cardioselective receptor-blocking agent. Ophthalmic betaxolol has minimal pul-

monary and cardiovascular side effects. Otherwise, this medication is contraindicated in patients who have sinus bradycardia, atrioventricular block that is greater than first-degree, cardiogenic shock, or overt cardiac failure.

d. Carbonic anhydrase inhibitors: carbonic anhydrase exists in the ciliary processes in the human eye. Carbonic anhydrase inhibitors have been found to lower intraocular pressure via a 50% to 60% reduction of aqueous humor formation. The diuretic effect of the carbonic anhydrase inhibitors is not a factor in the reduction of intraocular pressure.

(1) *Eyedrops*:

(a) *Dorzolamide HCl 2%*: dorzolamide HCl is a carbonic anhydrase inhibitor that decreases aqueous humor production by slowing the formation of bicarbonate ions with a consequent reduction in sodium and fluid transport. The result is a lowering of intraocular pressure.

(2) *Oral medications*:

(a) *Acetazolamide*: 250 mg every 6 hours by mouth (PO) or 500 mg sequels every 12 hours PO. Common side effects are paresthesias of the fingers, the toes, and the area around the mouth. Serum electrolyte imbalance can create metabolic acidosis from bicarbonate depletion. Potassium depletion may occur and may lead to significant hypokalemia in patients also taking chlorothiazide diuretics, digitalis, corticosteroids, or adrenocorticotropic hormone or in patients with hepatic cirrhosis. Renal calculi and, rarely, blood dyscrasias can occur.

(b) *Methazolamide*: 25 mg or 50 mg PO twice a day or 100 mg PO three times a day. A dose of 25 or 50 mg of methazolamide produces significant intraocular pressure reduction without causing metabolic acidosis.

E. Mydriatics and cycloplegics: these medications are used to dilate the pupil for diagnostic purposes. In eyes with narrow anterior chamber angles, these drops are used under the direction of an ophthalmologist. If these drops are improperly used in eyes with narrow anterior chamber angles, angle closure glaucoma can occur.

1. *Mydriatics (sympathomimetics)*.

a. *Phenylephrine HCl 2.5%*: this mydriatic dilates the pupil by stimulating the iris dilator muscle. It is used for the examination of the retina before cataract surgery and retinal procedures.

2. *Cycloplegics (parasympatholytics)*:

a. *Atropine sulfate 0.25%, 1%, 2%; ointment 0.5%, 1%*: this medication is used for cycloplegia, which is the paralysis of accommodation. The patient is unable to read printed material or see nearby objects. This temporary state enables the ophthalmologist to diagnose the need for spectacle correction in preverbal children. In the presence of acute inflammation and in the postoperative period, atropine may be used as well. In young children, toxic side effects can occur with excess use. The side effects include restlessness and excitatory behavior. Dry mouth, erythema of the face, absence of sweating, and tachycardia may occur.

b. *Cyclopentolate 0.5%, 1%, 2%*: this medication for cycloplegia is used for refraction in children and adults. In children, toxicity can be manifested by incoherence, visual hallucinations, slurred speech, and ataxia.

c. *Tropicamide 0.5%, 1%*: tropicamide has a greater mydriatic effect than a cycloplegic effect. Thus, it is used most often for mydriasis.

HOW TO READ AN OPHTHALMOLOGIST'S NOTE

V

(V = vision: top line is right eye [OD]; second line is the left eye [OS].)

T

(T = tension or intraocular pressure, measured in millimeters of mercury.)
(The top line is the right eye; the second line is the left eye.)

SLE

(SLE = slit lamp examination: used to evaluate the cornea, anterior chamber (AC), iris, lens.)

1. The cornea is described as "clear."
2. The anterior chamber is described as "deep and quiet" (D & Q) or as having "1+ to 4+ cells and/or flare (thick, viscous aqueous)."
3. The iris is described as being either blue or brown and with or without atrophy or rubeosis iridis.
4. The lens is described as having "1+ to 4+ nuclear sclerosis" (1+ to 4+ NS), a way to describe the amount of cataractogenesis present. Another way to characterize the lens is "1+ to 4+ cortical spokes," which describes the amount of opacity found in the lens. In a young person, the lens is described as being "clear."
5. The retina is described with respect to the optic disk, macula, vessels, equator, and periphery. Usually, a diagram accompanies this description.

COMMONLY PERFORMED TESTS IN THE OPHTHALMOLOGIST'S OFFICE

Fundus Photography and Slit Lamp Photography

Fundus photographs are useful for following the serial change in a patient's diabetic retinopathy, age-related macular degeneration, or other dynamic retinal changes. The photographs are useful for the recording of intraocular tumors, nevi, and growths. Slit-lamp photographs are useful for documenting abnormal lesions on the front of the eye. They are useful for recording conjunctival nevi or growths and for documenting trauma and for documenting trauma surgery before and after the procedure.

Fluorescein Angiography of the Fundus

Fluorescein angiography is used to document vascular lesions in the eye. It is commonly used for diabetic retinopathy, age-related macular degeneration, vascular occlusive disorders, tumors, vascular lesions, postoperative macular edema, and other abnormalities of the retina. It is used for diagnosis in inherited retinal dystrophies and viral disorders affecting the retina. Fluorescein angiography has a role in neovascular glaucoma. It has been used in infants and children with retinal disorders as well. Fluorescein angiography is useful in the preoperative evaluation for laser surgery.

Visual Field

The visual field is used to document visual loss. It serves to delineate peripheral visual field loss in glaucoma, altitudinal visual field loss in optic nerve disorders, and central nervous system disorders, and in nonspecific complaints of visual loss. It has been used in patients with headaches to diagnose transient scotomas. Four types of visual fields are used:
1. *Automated*: Used most commonly for glaucoma and testing of macular defects (Fig. AP–1).
2. *Goldmann*: Used for all visual field defects.
3. *Tangent screen*: Used to delineate the blind spot and altitudinal disorders in neurologic situations.
4. *Confrontational*: Used in an emergency department situation when more sophisticated testing is not immediately available. Confrontational visual fields can be very helpful in patients with neurologic dysfunction.

Testing of Eye Pressure

Schiøtz Tonometry. Measures the intraocular pressure by slightly indenting the cornea and measuring the resistance of the eye to the displacement of the volume. Its units are millimeters of mercury. Conversion tables are based on empirical data from in vivo and in vitro studies.

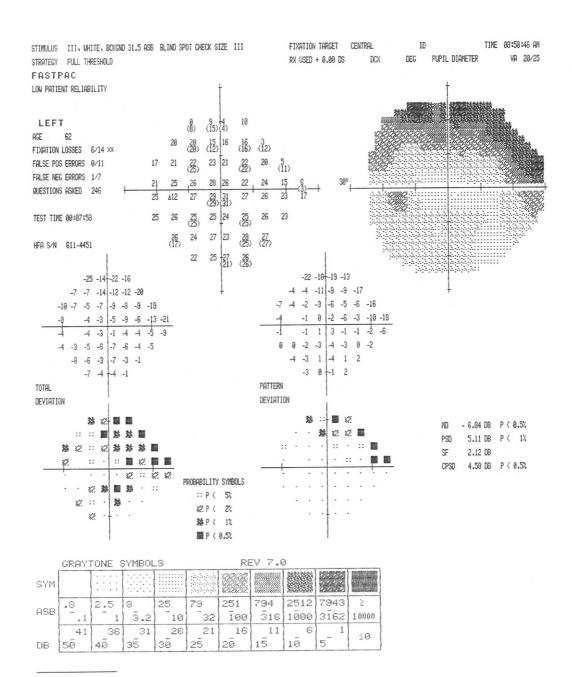

• **FIGURE AP-1**
Automated visual field.

Applanation Tonometry. Measures the intraocular pressure by slightly flattening the cornea and measures the force to flatten (applanate) a standard area of the corneal surface. The units are also in millimeters of mercury.

Provocative Testing for Glaucoma

Water Provocative Test. After an 8-hour fast, the test begins with a baseline applanation tonometry reading. The patient is instructed to drink 1 L of tap water, after which applanation is performed every 15 minutes for 1 hour. The maximum intraocular pressure increase usually occurs in 15 to 30 minutes after drinking the 1 liter of tap water and returns to the initial level after approximately 1 hour in both normal and glaucomatous eyes. A rise of 8 mm Hg is felt to be a significant response.

Dilation Provocative Test. Use of cycloplegic-mydriatic agents has been found to cause a significant pressure rise in certain eyes with open angle glaucoma. This test is useful in patients with exfoliation syndrome, pigmentary glaucoma, or open angle glaucoma with other causes of heavy pigmentation in the anterior chamber angle.

Evaluation of the Corneal Surface.

Keratometry is the measurement of the curvature of the cornea in the vertical and horizontal meridians. This technique is used to measure the size and power of the intraocular lens implant in cataract surgery. In addition, keratometry is used in the measurement for hard and soft contact lenses.

Corneal topography is the measurement of the corneal surface for its irregularities of curvature. This reading is used in the preoperative evaluation for the surgical correction of myopia.

Electroretinography

Electroretinography is the measurement of the retina's physiologic response to light, recorded in microvolts. The test has predictive value in diabetic retinopathy and neovascular glaucoma. Electroretinography plays a role in the diagnosis of rare, inherited retinal diseases and assesses the function of the retina in nonverbal individuals (Fig. AP–2).

Ultrasonography

Ultrasonography measures the axial length of the globe for cataract surgery. In addition, ultrasonography is used to visualize intraocular tumors,

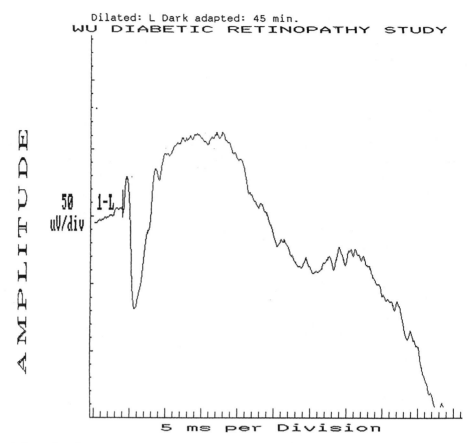

• FIGURE AP–2
Electroretinogram.

vitreous hemorrhage, or retinal detachment when the front of the eye is opaque to indirect and direct ophthalmoscopy.

Evaluation for Retinal Detachment and Fundus Drawing

This is used by ophthalmologists to map the retina in its entirety and to localize all of the pathology. Evaluation for retinal detachment and fundus drawing are useful for the clinical record, especially in patients with a history of retinal disease and in those who may undergo future surgery.

LASERS IN OPHTHALMOLOGY

A typical laser (light amplification by stimulated emission of radiation) has three parts: an *energy source*, a substance called the *active medium* and an *optical cavity* enclosing the active medium and two mirrors. One mirror reflects only part of the light striking it, and the other mirror is fully reflective. Stimulated emission occurs if atoms are in the excited state. An outside energy source pumps energy into the atoms and maintains them in the long-lived energy state. The mirrors in the active cavity reflect the photons back and forth in the active medium. The atoms are absorbing packets of light energy called *photons*. Each interaction of the photon and excited atom produces a chain reaction of stimulated emissions. This chain reaction causes a flood of light. All in phase, a strong beam of light called a *coherent beam of light* exits through a partly reflecting mirror.

Argon and Krypton Gas Lasers

The active medium is a gas or a mixture of gases in a tube. The atoms in gas lasers are excited by an electrical current. These are most commonly used for glaucoma and retinal problems. The amount of energy used is less than 1 W; the duration is usually 0.1 or 0.05 s. The spot size ranges from 50 to 500 μm. A larger spot size of 1000 μm can be used for specific retinal lesions. These lasers come in a large variety of wavelengths tailored to different pigmented lesions in the eye.

Diode Lasers

Diode lasers use semiconductors as the material that conducts the electricity. The junction between the layers serves as the active medium. When current flows across the junction, an overwhelming population of the atoms is in its excited state, thus producing a situation in which stimulated emission of photons can occur. The flat ends of the semiconductor serve as mirrors and internally reflect the photons, thus amplifying the light energy. The end result is the production of a coherent beam of light. These lasers are now being increasingly used for glaucoma and retinal problems. Their advantage is that these laser systems are portable and do not require an elaborate plumbing or electrical supply. Their disadvantage lies in their having fewer wavelength options.

Solid State Lasers

Solid state lasers use a rod made of solid material as the active medium. The most common crystal laser in ophthalmology contains the element neodymium (Nd) in an yttrium-aluminum-garnet (YAG) crystal. It produces laser light in pulses. It is used to treat postcataractous membrane growths in the eye.

Excimer Lasers

Excimer lasers use energy to create an "excited dimer" of rare gas and halide molecules in a gaseous cavity. In ophthalmology, argon fluoride gas is used. Then, pulses of ultraviolet light are released that are capable of removing layers of tissue from the cornea. This laser has its application in laser correction of myopia.

COMMON SURGICAL TECHNIQUES

Cataract Surgery

Cataract surgery is performed in a variety of methods at this writing.

The most common technique in patients with early-to-moderate cataracts is *phacoemulsification*, in which high-speed ultrasonic fragmentation is used to remove the lens nucleus. The capsular bag is left intact, and the plastic intraocular lens is inserted. All of this can be accomplished with a small incision in the sclera, sometimes necessitating one suture. The opening may be so small that no suture is needed to close the wound. In the case of very small wound openings, a foldable plastic lens is inserted.

Another common technique used in more mature and larger cataracts is called *extracapsular cataract extraction*, in which the lens nucleus is removed in toto and the nuclear bag is left in place. Then, the plastic intraocular lens implant is placed. The wound is usually larger than that in the phacoemulsification procedure described above.

In complicated cataracts involving retinal problems, the lens is removed with an ultrasonic fragmentation device placed in the same incisions as used for retinal surgery. This procedure is called *pars plana lensectomy* where the pars plana is the site of entrance for the instrument. The pars plana is the outermost extension of the retina.

Glaucoma Surgery

Glaucoma surgery is performed in those patients with severe glaucoma that is uncontrolled by medication, lasers, or other means. The principle involves placing another communicating channel for aqueous outflow.

A trabeculectomy can be used, in which a small opening is made in the trabecular meshwork and is covered by the conjunctiva. This is also called a filtering procedure. On occasion, the opening in trabeculectomy surgery is prematurely closed by overgrowth of abundant fibroblasts in the wound healing process. Thus, agents such as mitomycin C or 5 fluorouracil have been used to prolong the patency of the trabeculectomy site.

Other procedures involve placing a small narrow-lumen Silastic tube inside the anterior chamber; this tube drains the aqueous. The tube is connected to various plastic valve devices and is covered with a scleral patch graft. The entire prosthetic device is then covered by conjunctiva. This procedure is used in patients who have had previously unsuccessful surgical procedures.

Retinal Detachment Surgery

The simplest way to reattach the retina is by using soft plastic to support the wall of the sclera that corresponds to the area of detached retina. This operation is called a *scleral buckle*. It usually involves the use of laser or cryotherapy to ensure adhesion of the retina to the wall of the sclera.

More complicated procedures involve using instruments inside of the eye to remove scar tissue. This procedure is called a *vitrectomy* (removing the liquid vitreous). Mechanized cutting instruments are fitted inside a blunt needle, approximately the size of a 19-gauge needle. At the same time, the surgeon holds a light pipe, made of a fiberoptic cable, in the other hand. The third opening is for the infusion of balanced salt solution into the eye as the scar tissue or blood is removed.

Diabetic Eye Surgery

Using the aforementioned vitrectomy techniques, membrane peeling of the scar tissue is performed. Also, very commonly, blood inside the eye is removed. Laser photocoagulation is performed intraoperatively at this time as well.

Surgery for Trauma

Vitrectomy and scleral buckle procedures can be performed, depending on the difficulty of the case. Sometimes, the surgeon performs intraocular exploration for a foreign body. This process may entail the use of a magnet or other foreign body forceps to manipulate the safe removal of the foreign body.

Surgery for Myopia

Radial keratotomy is the flattening of the cornea by making radial incisions. This enables the light entering the cornea to bend and refract so that the light rays fall on the retina. This procedure can be performed by use of the excimer laser as well.

Optical Supply Companies

A. Topical eye drops, ointments, and related generic brand ophthalmic pharmaceutical products.
Akorn, Inc.
100 Akorn Drive
Abita Springs, LA 70420
Telephone: 800-535-7155

B. One of the original and largest ophthalmic pharmaceutical companies with national and international distribution networks. Has surgical instrumentation as well.
Alcon Ophthalmic
Alcon Laboratories, Inc.
Fort Worth, Texas 76134
Telephone: 800-451-3937

C. One of the largest ophthalmic pharmaceutical companies with national and international distribution networks. Has surgical instrumentation as well.
Allergan Pharmaceuticals, Inc.
Corporate Office
2525 Dupont Drive
P.O. Box 19534
Irvine, CA 92715
Telephone: 800-347-4500

D. Optical supply house selling E cards, Snellen charts, fluorescein strips, and related ophthalmic supplies and equipment.
Franklin Ophthalmic Instruments
12 Millville Road
Mendon, MA 01756
Telephone: 800-932-5083

E. Optical supply house selling E cards, Snellen charts, fluorescein strips, and related ophthalmic supplies and equipment.
Lombart Instruments
8676 Commerce Avenue
San Diego, CA 92121
Telephone: 800-446-8092

F. Optical supply house selling E cards, Snellen charts, fluorescein strips, and related ophthalmic supplies and equipment.
Lombart Instruments
5358 Robin Hood Road
Norfolk, VA 23513-2407
Telephone: 800-446-8092

G. Optical supply house selling E cards, Snellen charts, fluorescein strips, and related ophthalmic supplies and equipment.
Ophthalmic Instrument Company, Inc.
Avon Industrial Park
33 Wales Avenue
Avon, MA 02322
Telephone: 800-272-2070, 508-588-2070

Index

Page numbers in *italics* refer to illustrations; page numbers followed by t refer to tables. Color plate numbers are designated by CP preceding the number.

Abrasions, corneal, 50–51, *51*
Acetazolamide, for glaucoma, 181
Acquired immunodeficiency syndrome
    (AIDS), 125–130, *125–129*, 128t,
    CP 9–10
Acquired melanosis, 49
Active medium, in lasers, 187
Acuity, visual, 9, 10t, *11, 12*
Adie's pupil, 56. See also under Pupil(s).
Adnexa oculi, anatomy of, 3, *3, 4*, 4t
  disorders of, 25–31, *26–28*, 28t, 29t, *30*,
    30t
Adrenergic agents, for glaucoma, 180
Afferent pupillary defect, 55, *56–58*
AIDS (acquired immunodeficiency
    syndrome), 125–130, *125–129*, 128t,
    CP 9–10
Amblyopia, in children, 168–169
Angiography, fluorescein, 107–109, *109*
Angle, anatomy of, 5, *6*
Angle closure glaucoma, 79–81, 83t, 85–86,
    86, CP 4
Anterior chamber, anatomy of, 5
Anterior ischemic optic neuropathy,
    137–139, *138–139*, CP 11
Antibiotics, for eyes, 179
Applanation tonometry, 185
Aqueous fluid, 5
Argon lasers, 187
Arteritis, temporal, 139–142, *141*, CP 11
Artery, retinal. See *Retinal artery*.
Atropine sulfate, for glaucoma, 181–182
Automated tests, of visual field, 183, *184*

Bacitracin ophthalmic ointment, 179
Bacterial disease(s), conjunctivitis as, 47,
    47–48, CP 3
  keratitis as, 51
Basal cell carcinoma, of eyelid, 41, *42*,
    149–150, *150*, CP 2
Beta-adrenergic antagonists, for glaucoma,
    180–181
Betaxolol HCl, for glaucoma, 180–181
Blue dot hemorrhage, in diabetic
    retinopathy, 99, *102*, CP 7
Bowen's disease, 49
Buckle, scleral, 189

Cancer, 174. See also *Tumor(s)*; specific
    neoplasm.

Carbachol eyedrops, for glaucoma, 180
Carbonic anhydrase inhibitors, for
    glaucoma, 181
Carcinoma, of conjunctiva, 49, 152
  of eyelid, basal cell, 41, *42*, 149–150, *150*,
    CP 2
  squamous cell, 41, *42*, 150, *151*, CP 2
Cataracts, 59, *60*, 61–62, 61t, CP 3
  extracapsular, extraction of, 188
Cavity, optical, 187
Cellulitis, orbital, *28*, 28–29, CP 1
  preseptal, *27*, 27–28, CP 1
Chalazion, 25–27, *26*, 27t, CP 1
Child(ren), eye examination in, 161–169
    techniques of, 161t, 161–166, *162, 166*
  lazy eye in, 168–169
  ptosis in, 164
  strabismus in, 166–168, *167*
Choroid, anatomy of, 6, *6*
  melanoma of, 156–158, *156, 157*, CP 12
  tumors of, 154–156, *154, 155*, CP 12
Cicatricial entropion, 34
Cilia, 3, *3*
Ciliary body, anatomy of, 5, *6*
Ciprofloxacin hydrochloride eyedrops, 179
Closed-angle glaucoma, 79–81, 83t, 85–86,
    86, CP 4
Coherent beam of light, in lasers, 187
Confrontational tests, of visual field, 183
Congenital ptosis, 35–37, *36*, 164, *165*
Conjunctiva, anatomy of, 3, *3*
  Kaposi's sarcoma of, 127, *128*, CP 10
  nevus of, 47–49, *48*
  tumors of, *43*, 49–50, *50, 152*, 152–153
Conjunctivitis, bacterial, 47, *47–48*, CP 3
  herpes simplex, 45–46, 46t
  herpes zoster, 46, *47*, CP 2
  viral, 45, *45*, 46t
Contact lens, 22–25, 23t, *24*
  pain from, *87*, 87t, 87–88
Cornea, abrasions of, 50–51, *51*
  anatomy of, 3, *3*
  diabetes affecting, 112–113, 113t
  keratitis of, 51–52, *53*, 53t
  testing surface of, 185
  ulcers of, 52–53, 53t
Coronary artery disease, 174
Cotton wool spots, in AIDS, 125, *125*
  in diabetic retinopathy, 99, *101*, CP 7
Cyclopentolate, for glaucoma, 182
Cycloplegics, for glaucoma, 181–182
Cytomegalovirus retinitis, in AIDS,
    125–127, *126*, CP 9–10

Dacryocystitis, 29–31, *30*, 30t
Dermoid, 40, *41*
Detachment, retinal, 71–75, *71–74*, 75t, 186, 189, CP 4
Diabetic eye disease, corneal, 112–113, 113t
  disk swelling in, 144
  glaucoma as, 113–115, 113t–114t
  retinopathy as, 97–112, *97–110*, 104t–105t, 107t, CP 6
  review of systems in, 173–174
  surgery for, 189
Diclofenac sodium, for eyes, 179
Dilation provocative test, for glaucoma, 185
Diode lasers, 187
Dipivalyl epinephrine, for glaucoma, 180
Direct ophthalmoscope, in eye examination, 14–16, *15*
Dorzolamide HCl, for glaucoma, 181
Drugs, 179–182. See also specific drug.
Drusen, of optic disk, 142, *143*, CP 11
Dry eye, 54–55, 55t

E chart, 9, 10t, *11, 12*
Echothiophate eyedrops, for glaucoma, 180
Ectropion, 34t, 35, *35*
Edema, macular, 99, *100*, 104–106, *105*, 105t, 111, CP 8
  optic disk, 127–130, *129*, 142–146, *143*, CP 10–12
Electroretinography, 185, *186*
Embryology, of eye, 161
Emergencies, ophthalmic. See *Ophthalmic emergency(ies)*.
Energy source, in lasers, 187
Entropion, 33–35, *34*, 34t
Epinephrine HCl, for glaucoma, 180
Erythromycin ophthalmic ointment, 179
Excessive evaporation of tears, in dry eye, 54
Excimer lasers, 188
Extracapsular cataract extraction, 188
Exudates, hard, 99, *102*, CP 7
Eye. See also named parts of eye, e.g., *Cornea*.
  anatomy of, 3–6, *3, 4*, 4t, 5t, *6*
  disorder(s) of, cataracts as, 59, *60*, 61–62, 61t, CP 3
    chalazion as, 25–27, *26*, 27t, CP 1
    conjunctival, 45–50, *45*, 46t, *47–48, 50*
    contact lens overwear syndrome as, 22
    dacryocystitis as, 29–31, *30*, 30t
    diabetic retinopathy as, 97–112, *97–110*, 104t–105t, 107t, CP 6
    dry eye as, 54–55, 55t
    Graves' disease as, 31–33, *32*, 33t, CP 1
    hordeolum as, 25–27, *26*, 27t, CP 1
    hyperopia as, 19–21, *20*, 142
    inflammation as, 31–33, *32*, 33t, CP 1
    myopia as, 19, *20*, 189–190
    orbital cellulitis as, *28*, 28–29, CP 1
    presbyopia as, 21t, 21–22
    preseptal cellulitis as, *27*, 27–28, CP 1
  examination of, direct ophthalmoscope in, 14–16, *15*

Eye *(Continued)*
  fluorescein strips in, 14, *15*, CP 1
  frequency of, 9, 10t
  penlight in, 13–14, *14*
  pinhole in, 9–13, *13*
  visual acuity chart in, 9, 10t, *11, 12*
  medications for, 179–182
  pain in, 174–176
  trauma to, 88–94, *89–92*, 93t, *94*, CP 4–5
  tumors of. See *Tumor(s)*.
Eyeglasses, 22
Eyelid, carcinoma of, basal cell, 41, *42*, 149–150, *150*, CP 2
  sebaceous gland, 151
  squamous cell, 41, *42*, 150, *151*, CP 2
  ectropion of, 34t, 35, *35*
  entropion of, 33–35, *34*, 34t
  primary malignant tumors of, 149–151, *149–151*
  ptosis of, 35–37, *36*

Farsightedness, 19–21, *20*, 142
Fluorescein angiography, in diabetic retinopathy, 107–109, *109*
Fluorescein strips, in eye examination, 14, *15*, CP 1
Fluorometholone, for eyes, 179
Flurbiprofen sodium, for eyes, 179
Fundus, photography of, 182–183
  testing of, 186
Fungal keratitis, of cornea, 51–52, *53*

Gentamicin eyedrops, 179
Glaucoma, closed-angle, 79–81, 83t, 85–86, *86*, CP 4
  in diabetes, 113–115, 113t–114t
  medications for, 179–181
  neovascular, 114, *114*, 114t
  open-angle, 79, 81–85, *81, 82*, 83t, CP 4
  surgery for, 188–189
Goldmann tests, of visual field, 183
Graves' disease, 31–33, *32*, 33t, CP 1

Hard exudates, in diabetic retinopathy, 99, *102*, CP 7
Hemangioma, of conjunctiva, 49
Hemorrhage, blue dot, 99, *102*, CP 7
  in glaucoma, 114, *114*, 114t
  vitreous, 99, *101*, CP 6
Herpes simplex conjunctivitis, 45–46, 46t
Herpes simplex keratitis, 51–53, *52*, CP 3
Herpes zoster conjunctivitis, 46, *47*, CP 2
Hodgkin's lymphoma, *122*, 122–123
Hordeolum, 25–27, *26*, 27t, CP 1
Horner's syndrome, 57–58
Hyperopia, 19–21, *20*, 142
Hypertension, malignant, 144, *145*, CP 12
  review of systems in, 174

Hypertension *(Continued)*
 systemic, 115–118, *116*, 116t, *117*, 118t
Hypofunction, of lacrimal gland, 54

Inflammation, of eye, 31–33, *32*, 33t, CP 1
 of optic nerve, 134t, *136*, 136–137
Inhibitors, carbonic anhydrase, 181
Intraocular malignant melanoma, 43–44, *44*,
 CP 2
Iris, anatomy of, 3, *3*
Ischemic optic neuropathy, anterior,
 137–139, *138–139*, CP 11

Kaposi's sarcoma, in AIDS, 127, *128*, CP 10
Keratitis, of conjunctiva, 46, *47*, CP 2
 of cornea, bacterial, 51
  fungal, 51–52, *53*, 53t
  viral, 52, *53*, CP 3
Keratoacanthoma, 37–38, *38*, CP 2
Keratometry, in corneal surface testing, 185
Krypton gas lasers, 187

Lacrimal caruncle, anatomy of, 3, *4*
Lacrimal gland, hypofunction of, 54
Lasers, 109, *110*, CP 8
 coherent beam of light in, 187
 energy source in, 187
 photons in, 187
 solid state, 187–188
Lateral canthus, anatomy of, 3
"Lazy eye," in children, 168–169
Lens, anatomy of, 5–6, *6*. See also *Contact
 lens.*
Lensectomy, pars plana, in cataract surgery,
 188
Leukemia, 118–121, *119–120*, CP 9
Limbus, anatomy of, 3, *3*, 5t
Lymphoma, 41–43, *43*, 121–123, 152, CP 2
 Hodgkin's, *122*, 122–123
 non-Hodgkin's, 122, 122t, CP 9

Macroglobulinemia, 123
Macular edema, in diabetic retinopathy, 99,
 100, 104–106, *105*, 105t, 111, CP 8
Malignant hypertension, 144, *145*, CP 12
Marcus Gunn pupil, 55–56, *58*
Medial canthus, anatomy of, 3
Medications, 179–182. See also specific
 medication.
Medium, active, 187
Meibomian glands, orifices of, 3
Melanoma, intraocular malignant, 43–44,
 44, CP 2
 of choroid, 156–158, *156, 157*
 of conjunctiva, 48, 49–50, *50*, 152, CP 3,
  CP 12

Melanosis, acquired, 49
Metastatic disease, 122t, 123–125. See also
 Tumor(s); specific neoplasm.
Methazolamide, for glaucoma, 181
Microsurgery, in diabetic retinopathy,
 109–111
Milia, 37, *37*
Mucin deficiency, in dry eye, 54–55
Mydriatics, for glaucoma, 181–182
Myeloma, multiple, 123
Myopia, 19, *20*, 189–190

Nearsightedness, 19, *20*, 189–190
Necrosis, retinal, 127
Neoplasms. See *Tumor(s).*
Neovascular glaucoma, 114, *114*, 114t
Nerve, optic. See *Optic nerve.*
Neuritis, optic, 134t, *136*, 136–137
Neuropathy, optic, anterior ischemic,
 137–139, *138–139*, CP 11
Nevus(i), benign, 38, *39*, CP 1
 choroidal, *158*
 conjunctival, 47–49, *48*
Newborn, examination of, 163–164, *164*
 pseudoepicanthus in, 163, *164*
Non-diabetic retinopathy, 99, *103*, 104t,
 CP 6
Non-Hodgkin's lymphoma, 122, 122t, CP 9
Nonproliferative diabetic retinopathy, 104,
 104, CP 7
Nonsteroidal anti-inflammatory agents, for
 eyes, 179

Occlusion, retinal. See under *Retinal artery;
 Retinal vein.*
Ofloxacin 0.3% eyedrops, 179
Ointments, for eyes, 179, 180
Open-angle glaucoma, 79, 81–85, *81, 82*,
 83t, CP 4
Ophthalmia neonatorum, 163
Ophthalmic emergency(ies), chief complaint
 in, 173, 173t
 glaucoma as, 79–86, *80–82*, 83t, *84, 86*
 pain and contact lens use as, 87, 87t,
  87–88
 review of systems in, 173–174
 trauma as, 88–94, *89–92*, 93t, *94*, CP 4–5
Ophthalmologist, reading notes of, 182
 tests performed by, 182–188, *184, 186*
Ophthalmoscope, direct, 14–16, *15*
Optic disk, drusen of, 142, *143*, CP 11
 edema of, 127–130, *129*, 142–146, *143*,
  CP 10–12
Optic nerve, anatomy of, 6, *6*
 disorder(s) of, anterior ischemic optic neuropathy as, 137–139, *138–139*, CP 11
 hyperopia as, 19–21, *20*, 142
 inflammation as, 134t, *136*, 136–137
 malignant hypertension as, 144, *145*,
  CP 12

Optic nerve *(Continued)*
optic disk drusen as, 142, *143*, CP 11
papilledema as, *133*, 133–135, 134t, CP 10
papillitis as, 134t, 135–136
papillophlebitis as, 144–146, *145*, CP 12
pseudopapilledema as, 127–130, *129*, 142–146, *143*, CP 10–12
temporal arteritis as, 139–142, *141*, CP 11
venous stasis papillopathy as, 144–146, *145*, CP 12
Optical cavity, in lasers, 187
Orbit, anatomy of, 3, *3*
cellulitis of, *28*, 28–29, CP 1
tumors of, *149*, 153
Orifices, of meibomian glands, 3
Overwear syndrome, contact lens, 22

Pain, eye, 174–176
from contact lenses, *87*, 87t, 87–88
Papilledema, *133*, 133–135, 134t, CP 10
in AIDS, 127–130, *129*, CP 10
Papillitis, 134t, 135–136
Papilloma, 37, *37*
conjunctival, 49
Papillopathy, venous stasis, 144–146, *145*, CP 12
Papillophlebitis, 144–146, *145*, CP 12
Parasympathomimetic agents, for glaucoma, 180–182
Pars plana, 6, *71*, 71–72, 188, CP 4
Pediatric examination, 161–169
of newborn, 163–164, *164*
of premature infant, 164–166, *165, 166*
techniques of, 161t, 161–166, *162, 166*
Penlight, eye examination with, 13–14, *14*
Phacoemulsification, in cataract surgery, 188
Photons, in lasers, 187
Photography, of fundus, 182–183
slit lamp in, 182–183
Pilocarpine eyedrops, for glaucoma, 180
Pinhole, in eye examination, 9–13, *13*
Plica semilunaris conjunctiva, anatomy of, 3
Polymyxin B sulfate–bacitracin zinc ophthalmic ointment, 179
Prednisolone acetate, for eyes, 179
Prematurity, retinopathy of, 164–165, *165, 166*
Presbyopia, 21t, 21–22
Preseptal cellulitis, *27*, 27–28, CP 1
Pressure, eye, testing of, 183–185
Proliferative diabetic retinopathy, 106–107, 107t, *108*, 111, CP 8
Provocative testing, for glaucoma, 185
Pseudoepicanthus, in newborn, 163, *164*
Pseudopapilledema, 127–130, *129*, 142–146, *143*, CP 10–12
Ptosis, 35–37, *36*
congenital, 164, *165*
Pupil(s), Adie's, 56
afferent defect of, 55–56, *58*
examination of, 57t

Pupil(s) *(Continued)*
Horner's syndrome in, 57–58
unequal, 55
Pupillary light reflex, pathway of, *56*
Pupillary light test, *57*
Pupillary response, amaurotic, *59*

Retina, anatomy of, 6, *6*
detached, 71–75, *71–74*, 75t, 186, 189, CP 4
necrosis of, in AIDS, 127
tumors of, 154–156, *154, 155*, CP 12
Retinal artery, branch of, occlusion of, 65t, *70*, 70–71
central, occlusion of, 68–70, *69*
Retinal vein, branch of, occlusion of, 65t, *67*, 67–68, CP 3
central, occlusion of, 65–67, 65t, *66*, CP 3
Retinitis, cytomegalovirus, 125–127, *126*, CP 9–10
Retinoblastoma, 154–156, *154, 155*, CP 12
Retinopathy, diabetic, 97–112, *97–110*, 104t–105t, 107t, CP 6
hypertensive, 115–118, *116*, 116t, *117*, 118t
of prematurity, 164–165, *165, 166*
Rhabdomyosarcoma, of orbit, *149*, 153
Rimexolone, for eyes, 179

Sarcoma, Kaposi's, 127, *128*, CP 10
Schiøtz tonometry, 183
Sclera, anatomy of, 3
Scleral buckle, in retinal detachment surgery, 189
Sebaceous gland carcinoma, of eyelid, 151
Senile entropion, 33–34
Skin disorders, 25–31, *26–28*, 29t, *30*, 30t. See also specific disorder, e.g., *Cellulitis.*
Slit lamp photography, 182–183
Snellen visual acuity chart, 9, 10t, *11, 12*
Solid state lasers, 187–188
Squamous cell carcinoma, of eyelid, 41, *42*, 150, *151*, CP 2
Steroids, for eyes, 179
Strabismus, in children, 166–168, *167*
Strips, fluorescein, 14, *15*, CP 1
Sulfacetamide eyedrops, 179
Supply companies, 190–191
Surgery, 188–189
Systemic disease, acquired immunodeficiency syndrome as, 125–130, *125–129*, 128t, CP 9–10
diabetic retinopathy as, 97–112, *97–110*, 104t–105t, 107t, CP 6
dry eye as, 53–55, 55t
hypertension as, 115–118, *116*, 116t, *117*
leukemia as, 118–121, *119–120*, CP 9
lymphoma as, 41–43, *43*, 121–123, 122t, *122*, 152, CP 2, CP 9
metastatic, 122t, 123–125

Systemic disease *(Continued)*
  multiple myeloma as, 123
  of cornea, 112–113, 113t

Tangent screen tests, of visual field, 183
Tarsus, anatomy of, 3
Tears, excessive evaporation of, 54
Temporal arteritis, 139–142, *141*, CP 11
Testing, for glaucoma, 185
  of corneal surface, 185
  of fundus, 182–183, 186
  of retina, 185, 186, *186*
  of visual field, 183
Tetracycline ophthalmic ointment, 179
Timolol maleate, for glaucoma, 180
Tobramycin eyedrops, 179
Tonometry, 183–185
  applanation, 185
  Schiøtz, 183
Topography, corneal, 185
Trabecular meshwork, anatomy of, 5
Trabeculectomy, in glaucoma, 188–189
Trauma, to eye, 88–94, *89–92*, 93t, *94*,
    CP 4–5
  pain in, 174–176
  surgery for, 189
Tropicamide, for glaucoma, 182
Tumor(s), benign, dermoid as, 40, *41*
    keratoacanthoma as, 37–38, *38*, CP 2
    milia as, 37, *37*
    nevus as, 38, *39*, CP 1
    papilloma as, 37, *37*
    xanthelasma as, 38, *40*
  malignant, basal cell carcinoma as, 41, *42*,
      CP 2
    lymphoma as, 41–43, *43*, CP 2
    melanoma as, 43–44, *44*, CP 2
    squamous cell carcinoma as, 41, *42*,
        150, *151*, CP 2

Tumor(s) *(Continued)*
  of conjunctiva, *43*, 49–50, *50, 43, 152*,
      152–153
  of eyelids, 149–151, *149–151*
  of orbit, *149*, 153
  of retina and choroid, 153–155, *154, 155*,
      CP 12

Ulcers, of cornea, 52–53, 53t
Ultrasonography, 109, *110*, 185–186, CP 8
Unequal pupils, 55

Vein, retinal. See *Retinal vein.*
Venous stasis papillopathy, 144–146, *145*,
    CP 12
Viral conjunctivitis, 45, *45*, 46t
Viral keratitis, of cornea, 52, *53*, CP 3
Visual acuity, 9, 10t, *11, 12*
Visual field, testing of, 183, *184*
Vitrectomy, in retinal detachment surgery,
    189
Vitreous hemorrhage, in diabetic
    retinopathy, 99, *101*, CP 6

Water provocative test, for glaucoma, 185

Xanthelasma, 38, *40*

Zonules, anatomy of, 6, *6*